Conducting and Interpreting Clinical Trials in Heart Failure

Guest Editors

CHRISTOPHER M. O'CONNOR, MD
MONA FIUZAT, PharmD

HEART FAILURE CLINICS

www.heartfailure.theclinics.com

Consulting Editors
RAGAVENDRA R. BALIGA, MD, MBA
JAMES B. YOUNG, MD

Founding Editor
JAGAT NARULA, MD, PhD

October 2011 • Volume 7 • Number 4

Printed in the United States of America.

SAUNDERS an imprint of ELSEVIER, Inc.

W.B. SAUNDERS COMPANY
A Division of Elsevier Inc.

1600 John F. Kennedy Boulevard • Suite 1800 • Philadelphia, Pennsylvania 19103-2899

http://www.theclinics.com

HEART FAILURE CLINICS Volume 7, Number 4
October 2011 ISSN 1551-7136, ISBN-13: 978-1-4557-1102-4

Editor: Barbara Cohen-Kligerman
Developmental Editor: Donald Mumford

Heart Failure Clinics (ISSN 1551-7136) is published quarterly by Elsevier Inc., 360 Park Avenue South, New York, NY 10010-1710. Months of publication are January, April, July, and October. Business and editorial offices: 1600 John F. Kennedy Boulevard, Suite 1800, Philadelphia, PA 19103-2899. Periodicals postage paid at New York, NY, and additional mailing offices. Subscription prices are USD 207.00 per year for US individuals, USD 326.00 per year for US institutions, USD 70.00 per year for US students and residents, USD 248.00 per year for Canadian individuals, USD 374.00 per year for Canadian institutions, USD 264.00 per year for international individuals, USD 374.00 per year for international institutions, and USD 89.00 per year for Canadian and foreign students/residents. To receive student and resident rate, orders must be accompanied by name of affiliated institution, date of term, and the *signature* of program/residency coordinator on institution letterhead. Orders will be billed at individual rate until proof of status is received. Foreign air speed delivery is included in all *Clinics* subscription prices. All prices are subject to change without notice. **POSTMASTER:** Send address changes to *Heart Failure Clinics*, Elsevier Health Sciences Division, Subscription Customer Service, 3251 Riverport Lane, Maryland Heights, MO 63043. **Customer Service: 1-800-654-2452 (US and Canada). From outside of the US and Canada, call 314-447-8871. Fax: 314-447-8029. For print support, e-mail: JournalsCustomerService-usa@elsevier.com. For online support, e-mail: JournalsOnlineSupport-usa@elsevier.com.**

Reprints. For copies of 100 or more of articles in this publication, please contact the Commercial Reprints Department, Elsevier Inc., 360 Park Avenue South, New York, NY 10010-1710. Tel.: 212-633-3812; Fax: 212-462-1935; E-mail: reprints@elsevier.com.

Heart Failure Clinics is covered in *MEDLINE/PubMed (Index Medicus)*.

Printed and bound by CPI Group (UK) Ltd, Croydon, CR0 4YY

Transferred to Digital Print 2011

Cover artwork courtesy of Umberto M. Jezek.

Contributors

CONSULTING EDITORS

RAGAVENDRA R. BALIGA, MD, MBA
Vice-Chief and Assistant Division Director, Professor of Medicine, Division of Cardiovascular Medicine, The Ohio State University Medical Center, Columbus, Ohio

JAMES B. YOUNG, MD
Professor of Medicine and Executive Dean, Cleveland Clinic Lerner College of Medicine; George and Linda Kaufman Chair, Chairman, Endocrinology and Metabolism Institute, Cleveland Clinic, Cleveland, Ohio

GUEST EDITORS

CHRISTOPHER M. O'CONNOR, MD
Professor of Medicine; Director, Duke Heart Center; Acting Chief, Division of Cardiology; Chief, Division of Clinical Pharmacology, Duke University Medical Center, Durham, North Carolina

MONA FIUZAT, PharmD
Assistant Professor of Medicine, Duke University Medical Center, Durham, North Carolina

AUTHORS

PATRICIA A. ADAMS, BSN, RN
Lead Clinical Research Coordinator, Heart Failure Research, Duke University, Durham, North Carolina

SUZANNE ADAMS, RN, MPH
Manager, Division of Cardiology, Clinical Outcomes Research and Education, Jefferson Coordinating Center for Clinical Research, Jefferson Medical College, Jefferson Heart Institute, Philadelphia, Pennsylvania

LARRY A. ALLEN, MD, MHS
Assistant Professor of Medicine, Colorado Cardiovascular Outcomes Research Consortium, Section of Advanced Heart Failure, Division of Cardiology, Department of Medicine, University of Colorado Denver, Aurora, Colorado

LUCA BETTARI, MD
Duke Clinical Research Institute, Durham, North Carolina

RAPHAEL E. BONITA, MD, ScM
Assistant Professor of Medicine, Division of Cardiology, Jefferson Medical College, Philadelphia, Pennsylvania

SALVADOR BORGES-NETO, MD, FACC, FAHA, FACNP
Division of Cardiology, Duke University Medical Center, Durham, North Carolina

REBECCA BOXER, MD
Harrington McLaughlin Heart and Vascular Institute, Case Medical Center, University Hospitals of Cleveland, Cleveland, Ohio

MICHAEL R. BRISTOW, MD, PhD
Founder and CEO, ARCA Biopharma, Professor of Medicine, Division of Cardiology, University of Colorado Health Sciences Center, Denver, Colorado

ROBERT M. CALIFF, MD
Professor of Medicine, Director, Duke
Translational Medicine Institute; Vice
Chancellor for Clinical Research, Duke
University Medical Center and Duke
Translational Medicine Institute, Durham,
North Carolina

ZUBIN J. EAPEN, MD
Fellow, Department of Medicine, Duke Clinical
Research Institute, Duke University School
of Medicine, Durham, North Carolina

GREGORY EGNACZYK, MD, PhD
Division of Cardiology, Duke University
Medical Center, Durham, North Carolina

G. MICHAEL FELKER, MD, MHS
Associate Professor of Medicine, Duke Clinical
Research Institute, Durham, North Carolina

MONA FIUZAT, PharmD
Assistant Professor of Medicine,
Duke University Medical Center, Durham,
North Carolina

MIHAI GHEORGHIADE, MD
Professor of Medicine and Surgery,
Department of Medicine, Center for
Cardiovascular Innovation, Northwestern
University Feinberg School of Medicine,
Chicago, Illinois

ROBERT J. MENTZ, MD
Division of Cardiology, Department of
Medicine, Duke University Medical Center,
Durham, North Carolina

CARMELO A. MILANO, MD
Associate Professor of Surgery, Division
of Cardiothoracic Surgery, Duke University
Medical Center, Durham, North Carolina

CHRISTOPHER M. O'CONNOR, MD
Professor of Medicine; Director, Duke Heart
Center; Acting Chief, Division of Cardiology;
Chief, Division of Clinical Pharmacology,
Duke University Medical Center, Durham,
North Carolina

GERARD OGHLAKIAN, MD
Harrington McLaughlin Heart and Vascular
Institute, Case Medical Center, University
Hospitals of Cleveland, Cleveland, Ohio

PETER S. PANG, MD
Associate Professor of Emergency Medicine,
Department of Emergency Medicine,
Northwestern University Feinberg School
of Medicine; Assistant Professor of Medicine,
Department of Medicine, Center for
Cardiovascular Innovation, Northwestern
University Feinberg School of Medicine,
Chicago, Illinois

ILEANA L. PIÑA, MD, MPH
Professor of Medicine and Epidemiology/
Biostatistics, Case Western Reserve
University, Cleveland, Ohio

SHELBY D. REED, PhD
Associate Professor, Department of Medicine,
Duke Clinical Research Institute, Duke
University School of Medicine, Durham,
North Carolina

JOSEPH G. ROGERS, MD
Associate Professor of Medicine, Division
of Cardiology, Duke Clinical Research Institute,
Duke University Medical Center, Durham,
North Carolina

KEVIN A. SCHULMAN, MD
Professor, Department of Medicine, Duke
Clinical Research Institute, Duke University
School of Medicine, Durham, North Carolina

DAVID J. WHELLAN, MD, MHS
Director, Associate Professor of Medicine,
Division of Cardiology, Department of
Medicine, Clinical Outcomes Research and
Education, Jefferson Coordinating Center for
Clinical Research, Jefferson Medical College,
Jefferson Heart Institute, Thomas Jefferson
University, Philadelphia, Pennsylvania

Contents

Hospitalization for acute heart failure syndromes (AHFS) is a growing health care burden. Over 1 million hospitalizations occur annually, with a postdischarge mortality and rehospitalization rate of ~45% by 90 days and a financial cost greater than $20 billion. Attempts to improve outcomes through novel therapies have largely failed, suggesting new approaches are needed. We review phase II studies in AHFS to identify opportunities for future development programs.

Phase 3 clinical trials in acute heart failure are conducted to allow safety and efficacy data to be collected for the evaluation of treatment strategies, including drugs, devices, diagnostics, or nonpharmacological interventions. There are several important features regarding the conduct of phase 3 clinical trials in acute heart failure. This article describes in detail these important aspects of conducting phase 3 clinical trials in an acute heart failure population.

Recent advances in mechanically assisted circulation, including refinement of patient selection criteria and enhancements in device design, have been associated with improvements in survival, functionality and quality of life as well as reductions in adverse events. Novel and innovative trial design, methodology and endpoints have been utilized in the development of the cumulative database supporting the role of ventricular assist devices for the management of patients with advanced heart failure. The rapid and significant improvements in patient-centric outcomes support the expansion of this technology into less moribund populations where the potential benefits may be even more robust.

With the aging of the population and advances in acute treatment of ischemic events and surgical techniques for coronary artery and valvular heart disease, the prevalence of heart failure has been increasing. Lifestyle modifications are an integral part of preventing and treating most pathologic human conditions, and include behavioral modifications, diet, and exercise. Despite advances in medical and device therapy for heart failure, clinicians still hope that patients will adhere to nonpharmacologic interventions, some of which can actually improve symptoms and quality of life. This article reviews the role of these lifestyle modifications in preventing and treating heart failure.

Part II. Endpoints and Methodological Considerations

The appropriate selection of response variables for clinical trials of new therapies for acute heart failure (AHF) is a complex process with major trade-offs. For one therapeutic approach to be considered superior to another, it must produce clinically significant improvements in making patients live longer, making patients feel better, or saving resources without adversely affecting these two goals. This review outlines factors that complicate AHF end-point selection, discusses a variety of end points used in recently completed and ongoing AHF studies, and suggests directions for future design and standardization of end points across AHF trials.

Randomized controlled clinical trials are predominantly used to determine the benefit of a therapeutic intervention in patients with congestive heart failure (HF). These trials are commonly lengthy and expensive, and enroll patients with baseline imbalances that may influence outcome, even after randomization. Methods allowing for greater precision, power, and adjustment for treatment effect would be welcomed. Covariate adjustment may provide more individualized effect estimates and a potential improvement in power and reduction in type 1 error. This article reviews the HF-ACTION trial to better understand whether covariate adjustment should be prespecified as the primary end point in HF clinical trials.

Despite the continued growth of heart failure as a major public health problem, the development of new therapies for heart failure has slowed and recent studies have been neutral, suggesting the need for a reappraisal of the clinical research enterprise. Surrogate end points, defined as measurements that are used as substitutes for the more clinically meaningful end points, can play a valuable role in clinical trials by accelerating the timeline for determining appropriate dosages, efficacy, and safety. Biomarkers, such as the natriuretic peptides, have many of the characteristics of valid surrogates but have not been sufficiently validated for widespread use. Ongoing research into the role of biomarkers as surrogates may lead to better clinical trial design and more efficient development of new therapies for heart failure.

Despite the epidemiologic importance, large investments, and careful design, recent results of heart failure (HF) trials have been unable to demonstrate significant treatment improvements. This shortcoming has led to a reassessment of research methodology, particularly related to sample size and costs, for which end-point selection is a main issue. In comparing interventions in clinical trials, surrogate end points may be used to reduce the costs. To this end, ongoing research into the roles of imaging biomarkers as reliable surrogate end points may lead to better clinical trial design and more efficient development of new therapies for HF.

Cardiorenal syndrome is a focus of interest in heart failure because of the substantial associated morbidity and mortality. Recent clinical trials of novel heart failure therapies targeting the interdependence of cardiac and renal dysfunction have failed to show significant benefits with respect to many end points. The heterogeneity of this patient population and the lack of standardized clinical trial end points complicate forward progress. This article reviews the end points evaluated in key clinical trials of cardiorenal syndrome and synthesizes recent discussions about the appropriateness of end points for future trials.

The selection of economic end points in acute decompensated heart failure (ADHF) clinical trials requires prospectively planned evaluations that are developed in tandem with clinical end points. Integrating economic end points with concrete clinical outcomes postdischarge will provide meaningful data to evaluate a treatment's incremental value in the setting of ADHF.

Part III. Special Topics

Clinical trials are often conducted globally. Differences in standard of care, patient populations including genetic and phenotypic differences, disease etiologies, rates of comorbidities, ascertainment of endpoints, and differences in concomitant therapies and medical culture may influence subsequent outcomes. There has been little consensus on how clinical trial results should be evaluated. This article reviews the differences in cardiovascular trial results by geographic region, offers potential explanations for these differences, and suggests methods for standardization of trial results.

The conduct of clinical trials in acute heart failure has arrived at a critical point. Traditional systems used to conduct clinical trials have been described as inefficient, lacking infrastructure, and enormously expensive. In this article, the authors describe an alternative model: the development of a site-based research (SBR) unit, an operating business unit responsible for conducting a portfolio of research projects in a therapeutic area. The SBR is responsible for financial accountability, regulatory compliance, and academic productivity.

Pharmacogenetics in Heart Failure Trials

Mona Fiuzat and Michael R. Bristow

> There is ongoing research into potential pharmacogenetic targets in heart failure. Several challenges exist despite the potential benefits, and questions remain on the level of evidence needed to support product approval or labeling. High annual mortality, high morbidity, and heterogeneity of response to treatment underscore the need for predictability of response in this patient population. Although prime time testing and application of pharmacogenetics is not currently being used in heart failure, we believe this treatment approach is not too distant. The data are supportive, and further research is warranted to strengthen the approach.

Reporting of Clinical Trials: Publication, Authorship, and Trial Registration

Raphael E. Bonita, Suzanne Adams, and David J. Whellan

> Transparency is the foundation on which all of research integrity rests. The public trust from patients, providers, and policy makers depends on fidelity to the mandates of accountability and access. Two important foundational practices for maintaining transparency in research and the reporting of clinical trials discussed in this review concern manuscript authorship and clinical trial registry, recognizing recent controversies regarding honorary and ghost authorship in the publication of industry-sponsored studies.

Heart Failure Clinics

VISIT THE CLINICS ONLINE!

Access your subscription at:
http://www.theclinics.com

Editorial

Clinical Trials to "Real-World" Heart Failure: Applying Risk Stratification to Deliver Personalized Care

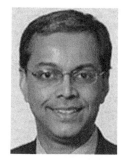 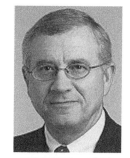

Ragavendra R. Baliga, MD, MBA   James B. Young, MD

Consulting Editors

Randomized clinical trials have resulted in rapid advances in the management of heart failure[1] in the last decade because of availability of neurohormonal modulating agents, including angiotensin receptor and converting enzyme inhibitors[2–7]; β-blockers[8,9]; aldosterone receptor antagonists[10,11]; devices such as the implantable cardioverter-defibrillator; and heart failure–specific disease management programs. Despite these rapid advances, the mortality rates in heart failure remain high even in very-low-risk patients, in whom the 5-year case fatality was 24% in a recently reported population-based study and the 5-year case fatality associated with a new admission for heart failure is close to 70%.[12] This rate is only marginally better than the 5-year case fatality of 75% reported in a comparable study covering a period between 1995 and 2000.

A meaningful impact on heart failure mortality requires a method that goes beyond the specific discrete interventional approach typically evaluated in randomized clinical trials. Randomized clinical trials are helpful in that they promote better understanding of the average overall benefit and risk of a particular therapy in a selected cohort of patients.[13] In the real-world situation, patients often have several comorbidities,[14] such as cardiorenal syndrome,[15] atrial fibrillation, chronic lung conditions, dyslipidemia, stroke, systolic blood pressure, dyslipidemia, and severity of systolic dysfunction that increase risk of mortality. These patients are frequently not included in clinical trials, which creates a clinical trial bias of ascertainment. Subsequently, such patients with the highest risk of mortality are less likely to receive optimal therapy even when they may be most likely to obtain the greatest absolute benefit with a specific therapy.[16]

For example, randomized clinical trials assessing the efficacy of spironolactone, β-blockers, or angiotensin-converting enzyme inhibitors generally excluded patients with azotemia,[17,18] who may have the highest heart failure mortality.[19] As a result, a large real-world population-based study found elevated serum potassium levels and increased mortality in patients treated with spironolactone.[20] These findings were attributed to the use of spironolactone in patients with greater risk of hyperkalemia than described in the randomized clinical trials. The cause of heart failure, age of the patient, hyponatremia, and elevated serum biomarker levels are other important factors that can influence overall prognosis. All these factors are also likely to influence choice of therapy, and a personalized approach in which treatments that are most likely to be beneficial to a given patient require taking all these risk factors into consideration (**Fig. 1**).

Heart Failure Clin 7 (2011) xi–xiv
doi:10.1016/j.hfc.2011.08.009

heartfailure.theclinics.com

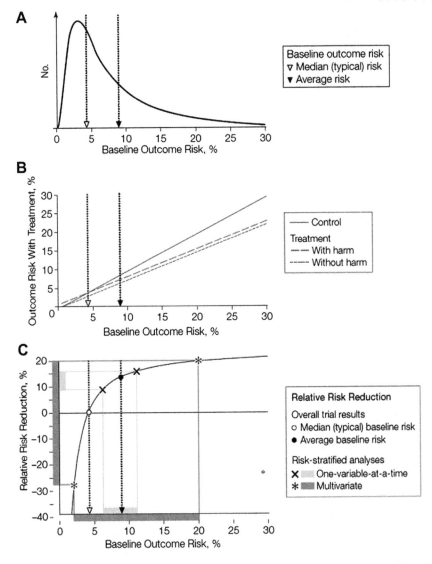

Fig. 1. Population distribution of baseline outcome risk, outcome risk with treatment, and relative risk reduction. (*From* Kent DM, Hayward RA. Limitations of applying summary results of clinical trials to individual patients: the need for risk stratification. JAMA 2007;298(10):1209–10; with permission.)

Risk-based analysis allows insight into the variation of therapeutic effect in patients who have multiple attributes that affect the likelihood of the outcome and the effect of therapy.[21] However, risk-based analysis is rarely performed in clinical trials, and, as a result, it remains unclear whether the summary results of a clinical trial actually apply to most of the patients in the trial.[21] A moderately predictive multivariate prediction tool should allow risk stratification because a multivariate risk–stratified model compares therapeutic effects across a broader spectrum of baseline risk (often ranging by 10–30 fold) as compared with a conventional one-variable-at-a-time subgroup analysis (few

independent risk factors increase risk by more than 2-fold).[21,22] The former approach should minimize shortcomings of the latter method, including false-positive and false-negative findings. In addition, a comprehensive risk model should include factors such as risk of treatment-related harm, risk of competing outcomes unresponsive to treatment, and factors that directly modify therapeutic effects.

At present, the American Heart Association/American College of Cardiology guidelines[23] continue to recommend management based on crude averages because of a paucity of consistent analytic approach that informs the practicing clinician how an individual patient's characteristics combine to affect the fundamental determinants of benefits of therapy versus the individual risk of poor outcomes in the absence of therapy versus the individual's risk of poor outcomes if treated, whereas the more recently reported National Institute for Health and Clinical Excellence guidelines attempt to risk stratify patients based on serum natriuretic peptide levels, echocardiography, and specialist assessment in the diagnosis of heart failure.[24]

Arguably, the multicenter, randomized, double-blinded megatrial has become the coin of the realm in determining so-called evidence-based therapies and thus treatment guidelines for patients with the broadly defined clinical heart failure. We must guard against undue intellectualization regarding this and particularly slavish worship of the P value. Further, we must improve the science and the art of the clinical trial so that we can help our patients more. Particularly important is using clinical trial (and registry) data to better predict individual responses to therapeutic maneuvers. We have come to an odd position where we simply add on another drug that has been proven effective by clinical trials using the group mean model, as discussed. One might wonder about how many great therapies have been discarded because of clinical trial design limitations giving us the wrong answer for specific individuals who have become buried in the mass of group mean models. It is a fascinating and important challenge to address.

To discuss the benefits and limitations of randomized clinical trials Christopher O'Connor, MD, and Mona Fizuat, PharmD, from Duke University have put together an international panel of experts. In our opinion an individualized approach using multivariate risk analysis based on readily obtainable real-world clinical attributes should be routinely performed to make further reductions in mortality due to heart failure to decrease length of stay and reduce rehospitalization rates.[25]

Ragavendra R. Baliga, MD, MBA
Division of Cardiovascular Medicine
The Ohio State University Medical Center
Columbus, OH, USA

James B. Young, MD
Lerner College of Medicine
Endocrinology & Metabolism Institute
Cleveland Clinic
Cleveland, OH, USA

E-mail addresses:
Ragavendra.baliga@osumc.edu (R.R. Baliga)
youngj@ccf.org (J.B. Young)

REFERENCES

1. Young JB. Clinical trials with implications regarding heart failure therapy. Curr Opin Cardiol 1997;12(4): 407–17.
2. Cohn JN, Johnson G, Ziesche S, et al. A comparison of enalapril with hydralazine-isosorbide dinitrate in the treatment of chronic congestive heart failure. N Engl J Med 1991;325(5):303–10.
3. Davis R, Ribner HS, Keung E, et al. Treatment of chronic congestive heart failure with captopril, an oral inhibitor of angiotensin-converting enzyme. N Engl J Med 1979;301(3):117–21.
4. Inhibition of angiotensin-converting enzyme in congestive heart failure. N Engl J Med 1987;316(14): 879–80.
5. Effects of enalapril on mortality in severe congestive heart failure. Results of the Cooperative North Scandinavian Enalapril Survival Study (CONSENSUS). The CONSENSUS Trial Study Group. N Engl J Med 1987;316(23):1429–35.
6. Effect of enalapril on survival in patients with reduced left ventricular ejection fractions and congestive heart failure. The SOLVD Investigators. N Engl J Med 1991;325(5):293–302.
7. Effect of enalapril on mortality and the development of heart failure in asymptomatic patients with reduced left ventricular ejection fractions. The SOLVD Investigators. N Engl J Med 1992;327(10):685–91.
8. Packer M, Bristow MR, Cohn JN, et al. The effect of carvedilol on morbidity and mortality in patients with chronic heart failure. U.S. Carvedilol Heart Failure Study Group. N Engl J Med 1996;334(21):1349–55.
9. Packer M, Coats AJ, Fowler MB, et al. Effect of carvedilol on survival in severe chronic heart failure. N Engl J Med 2001;344(22):1651–8.
10. Zannad F, McMurray JJ, Krum H, et al. Eplerenone in patients with systolic heart failure and mild symptoms. N Engl J Med 2011;364(1):11–21.
11. Pitt B, Zannad F, Remme WJ, et al. The effect of spironolactone on morbidity and mortality in patients with severe heart failure. Randomized Aldactone Evaluation Study Investigators. N Engl J Med 1999;341(10):709–17.
12. Bui AL, Horwich TB, Fonarow GC. Epidemiology and risk profile of heart failure. Nat Rev Cardiol 2011; 8(1):30–41.
13. Rothwell PM. External validity of randomised controlled trials: "to whom do the results of this trial apply?" Lancet 2005;365(9453):82–93.
14. Charlson ME, Pompei P, Ales KL, et al. A new method of classifying prognostic comorbidity in longitudinal studies: development and validation. J Chronic Dis 1987;40(5):373–83.
15. Baliga RR, Young JB. Staying in the pink of health for patients with cardiorenal anemia requires a multidisciplinary approach. Heart Fail Clin 2010;6(3):xi–xvi.

16. Lee DS, Tu JV, Juurlink DN, et al. Risk-treatment mismatch in the pharmacotherapy of heart failure. JAMA 2005;294(10):1240–7.

17. Coca SG, Krumholz HM, Garg AX, et al. Underrepresentation of renal disease in randomized controlled trials of cardiovascular disease. JAMA 2006;296(11): 1377–84.

18. Shlipak MG. Pharmacotherapy for heart failure in patients with renal insufficiency. Ann Intern Med 2003;138(11):917–24.

19. McAlister FA, Ezekowitz J, Tonelli M, et al. Renal insufficiency and heart failure: prognostic and therapeutic implications from a prospective cohort study. Circulation 2004;109(8):1004–9.

20. Juurlink DN, Mamdani MM, Lee DS, et al. Rates of hyperkalemia after publication of the Randomized Aldactone Evaluation Study. N Engl J Med 2004; 351(6):543–51.

21. Kent DM, Hayward RA. Limitations of applying summary results of clinical trials to individual patients: the need for risk stratification. JAMA 2007;298(10): 1209–12.

22. Hayward RA, Kent DM, Vijan S, et al. Multivariable risk prediction can greatly enhance the statistical power of clinical trial subgroup analysis. BMC Med Res Methodol 2006;6:18.

23. Hunt SA, Abraham WT, Chin MH, et al. 2009 Focused update incorporated into the ACC/AHA 2005 Guidelines for the Diagnosis and Management of Heart Failure in Adults A Report of the American College of Cardiology Foundation/American Heart Association Task Force on Practice Guidelines Developed in Collaboration With the International Society for Heart and Lung Transplantation. J Am Coll Cardiol 2009; 53(15):e1–90.

24. Mant J, Al-Mohammad A, Swain S, et al. Management of chronic heart failure in adults: synopsis of the National Institute for Health and Clinical Excellence Guideline. Ann Intern Med 2011;155(4): 252–9.

25. Smith DH, Johnson ES, Thorp ML, et al. Integrating clinical trial findings into practice through risk stratification: the case of heart failure management. Popul Health Manag 2010;13(3):123–9.

Preface

Clinical Trials in Acute Decompensated Heart Failure—Over 50 Years of Research

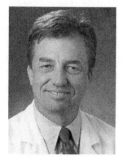 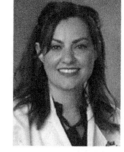

Christopher M. O'Connor, MD   Mona Fiuzat, PharmD

Guest Editors

This issue of *Heart Failure Clinics* is dedicated to an in-depth analysis of the conduct of clinical investigation in patients with acute decompensated heart failure (ADHF). We would like to start with a reflection on the history of ADHF research over the past 50 years.

For many years, ADHF was thought to be a temporary inconvenience in the course of the chronic heart failure patient, in which a short-term disturbance resulted in a need for intravenous therapies, subsequent hospitalization, and a return to baseline. It was not until the observations from the OPTIME trial that we found an extraordinarily high rate of readmission and death at 60 days in these patients.[1] This heightened risk of morbidity and mortality led us to believe that this was a very important condition that required in-depth attention and investigation.

Before the completion of the OPTIME trial in 2002, much of our reasoning for the goal of intervention was based on physiologic response. For example, some of the first articles described by Dr Eugene Stead offered insight into the important complex interaction between the heart and kidney in heart failure patients.[2] Dr Walter Kempner further elaborated on this complex interaction between the heart and kidney by demonstrating that significant sodium restriction could result in improvement in the clinical edematous state and improvement in the symptoms of heart failure patients.[3] Dr Stead went on to describe further the importance of vasopressin and the role of fluid retention in the heart failure patient, elaborating on the interaction between the heart and kidney.[4] During this time period, there were enormous contributions to the observation that hemodynamics were significantly disturbed, and the decompensated heart failure patient was characterized by increased filling pressures and reduced cardiac index. Further, we learned that decompensation also resulted in deterioration of right ventricular function and elevated pulmonary artery pressures.[5–8]

Continued observations were made throughout the 1960s, 1970s, and 1980s by Dr Eugene Braunwald[9] and others, on the role of hemodynamics, neurohormonal activation, peripheral adaptation and exercise intolerance for the explanation of fatigue in these patients.[10] Dr Joseph Greenfield went on to describe the importance of coronary blood flow in the ischemic etiology of heart failure.[11] Early observations highlighted the importance of neurohormonal activation of the sympathetic nervous system and other systems contributing to the progression of disease and mortality, leading investigators to take alternative approaches to the hemodynamic model of targeting therapy in patients with ADHF.[12–15]

Heart Failure Clin 7 (2011) xv–xvii

doi:10.1016/j.hfc.2011.06.015

heartfailure.theclinics.com

Surprisingly, in the 1960s, the first study of vasodilator therapy in acute heart failure after myocardial infarction showed that nitroprusside indeed could be harmful when administered early in this population.[16] In the 1980s, intravenous milrinone was approved for the treatment of heart failure in hospitalized heart failure patients on the basis of a relatively small patient safety database using hemodynamic endpoints. As the field evolved, it became clear that hemodynamic endpoints alone were not enough to guarantee safety or efficacy in patients who were receiving these therapies.

Two parallel programs resulted in observations described in 2002. One was the development of nesiritide, the beta-type receptor natriuretic peptide, which was developed to show improvement in hemodynamics similar to IV nitroglycerin and also was targeted to show a quicker and more sustained relief of dyspnea. The V-MAC study was the first to show that an intravenous therapy for heart failure demonstrated an improvement in symptoms above and beyond hemodynamics, which led to the approval of this therapy.[17]

Simultaneous with the publication of V-MAC was the publication of the OPTIME study, which enrolled 986 patients and was the largest study of ADHF to date.[1] Intravenous milrinone was tested against usual care with the clinically meaningful endpoint of total days alive and out of the hospital at 60 days, as well as other clinical endpoints. Surprisingly, intravenous milrinone showed no advantage to usual care in this population and was associated with more serious adverse cardiovascular events. Thus, during this time, the role of routine inotropic therapy in ADHF patients was questioned, and its use diminished to less than 10% of patients presenting with ADHF. On the other hand, the vasodilator strategy became highly popular and deployed by clinicians.

At the same time, however, the intravenous prostacyclin study of Flolan in advanced heart failure was conducted (FIRST-HF).[18] This pure vasodilator, when compared to usual care in a double-blind placebo-controlled study, showed no advantage on clinical outcomes of morbidity and mortality despite showing an advantage in acute hemodynamic effect. Again, this led investigators to question whether targeting pure hemodynamics, as opposed to hemodynamics plus neurohormonal modulation, was the proper target for investigation.

A series of therapies targeted toward the neurohormonal axis proved to be disappointing in improving clinical outcomes. These included the intravenous endothelin antagonists, vasopressin antagonists, cytokine modulators, and adenosine A1 antagonists.[19–22] Although disappointing, the robustness of the clinical design of these trials focusing on clinical endpoints allowed the field to mature and allowed us to better understand the patient population, clinical course, and challenges of improving outcomes in these complex patients.

To this end, the ASCEND-HF trial finished with a remarkable enrollment of over 7000 patients, a sample size thought to be unachievable in this population.[23] With clinically meaningful endpoints of dyspnea and rehospitalization for heart failure or death at 30 days, this trial will stand as the landmark for the development of new interventions. It completes a complicated course for the drug nesiritide, which achieved improvement in dyspnea in a trial of 489 patients.[17] Subsequently, meta-analyses of several small trials showed safety concerns with renal function and mortality, forcing the academic community, with the support of the sponsor, to challenge the role of this drug by conducting a morbidity and mortality safety trial.[24]

With the ASCEND-HF trial, we have completed a 10-year evolution in the conduct of investigation in ADHF that started with using surrogate endpoints, such as hemodynamics, and small sample size trials—to finish with trials having sample sizes that are robust and rigorous and can stand the test of inquisition that parallel the field of acute coronary syndromes, which have been the basis for evidence-based outcomes trials in cardiology over the past three decades.

We are proud to dedicate this edition of *Heart Failure Clinics* to the design considerations of clinical trials in acute heart failure. We hope the information is meaningful and useful for thinking about the design of clinical trials in this field. We will take you on a journey from early phase studies through late phase studies and tackle the difficult questions involved in patient population, trial conduct, surrogate endpoints, clinical endpoints, and statistical considerations. Thank you and enjoy your learning.

Christopher M. O'Connor, MD
Division of Cardiology
Duke University Medical Center
DUMC 3356
Durham, NC 27710, USA

Mona Fiuzat, PharmD
Duke University Medical Center
2400 Pratt Street, Room 8011
Durham, NC 27710, USA

E-mail addresses:
oconn002@mc.duke.edu (C.M. O'Connor)
mona.fiuzat@duke.edu (M. Fiuzat)

REFERENCES

1. Cuffe MS, Califf RM, Adams KF Jr, et al. Short-term intravenous milrinone for acute exacerbation of chronic heart failure: a randomized controlled trial. JAMA 2002;287:1541–7.

2. Stead EA Jr. Renal factor in congestive heart failure. Circulation 1951;3:294–9.

3. Kempner W. Effect of salt restriction on experimental nephrosis. JAMA 1965;191:51.

4. Stead EA Jr. Edema and dyspnea of heart failure. Bull NY Acad Med 1952;28:159–67.

5. Gorlin R. Prevention of remodeling of the heart after myocardial infarction. Mt Sinai J Med 1995; 62:287–92.

6. Cobb FR, Bache RJ, Ebert PA, et al. Effects of beta-receptor blockade on the systemic and coronary hemodynamic response to an increasing ventricular rate in the unanesthetized dog. Circ Res 1969;25: 331–41.

7. Gorlin R, Warren JV. Hemodynamic methods: heart and lungs: introduction. Methods Med Res 1958;7: 60–1.

8. Guiha NH, Limas CJ, Cohn JN. Predominant right ventricular dysfunction after right ventricular destruction in the dog. Am J Cardiol 1974;33:254–8.

9. Braunwald E. Coronary artery spasm. Mechanisms and clinical relevance. JAMA 1981;246(17):1957–9.

10. Sonnenblick EH, Braunwald E, Williams JF Jr, et al. Effects of exercise on myocardial force-velocity relations in intact unanesthetized man: relative roles of changes in heart rate, sympathetic activity, and ventricular dimensions. J Clin Invest 1965;44:2051–62.

11. Greenfield JC Jr, Cox RL. Instantaneous pressure-flow-length relationships in the intact human heart. Am J Med Sci 1968;255:288–91.

12. Bristow MR. The adrenergic nervous system in heart failure. N Engl J Med 1984;311:850–1.

13. Spann JF Jr, Sonnenblick EH, Cooper T, et al. Cardiac norepinephrine stores and the contractile state of heart muscle. Circ Res 1966;19:317–25.

14. Packer M. The neurohormonal hypothesis: a theory to explain the mechanism of disease progression in heart failure. J Am Coll Cardiol 1992;20:248–54.

15. Cohn JN. Comparative cardiovascular effects of tyramine, ephedrine, and norepinephrine in man. Circ Res 1965;16:174–82.

16. Guiha NH, Cohn JN, Mikulic E, et al. Treatment of refractory heart failure with infusion of nitroprusside. N Engl J Med 1974;291:587–92.

17. Publication Committee for the VMAC Investigators. Intravenous nesiritide vs nitroglycerin for treatment of decompensated congestive heart failure: a randomized controlled trial. JAMA 2002;287: 1531–40.

18. Califf RM, Adams KF, McKenna WJ, et al. A randomized controlled trial of epoprostenol therapy for severe congestive heart failure: The Flolan International Randomized Survival Trial (FIRST). Am Heart J 1997;134:44–54.

19. Moiseyev VS, Poder P, Andrejevs N, et al. Safety and efficacy of a novel calcium sensitizer, levosimendan, in patients with left ventricular failure due to an acute myocardial infarction. A randomized, placebo-controlled, double-blind study (RUSSLAN). Eur Heart J 2002;23:1422–32.

20. McMurray JJ, Teerlink JR, Cotter G, et al. Effects of tezosentan on symptoms and clinical outcomes in patients with acute heart failure: the VERITAS randomized controlled trials. JAMA 2007;298: 2009–19.

21. Mebazaa A, Nieminen MS, Packer M, et al. Levosimendan vs dobutamine for patients with acute decompensated heart failure: the SURVIVE Randomized Trial. JAMA 2007;297:1883–91.

22. Cleland JG, Freemantle N, Coletta AP, et al. Clinical trials update from the American Heart Association: REPAIR-AMI, ASTAMI, JELIS, MEGA, REVIVE-II, SURVIVE, and PROACTIVE. Eur J Heart Fail 2006; 8:105–10.

23. O'Connor CM, Starling RC, Hernandez AF, et al. Effect of nesiritide in patients with acute decompensated heart failure. N Engl J Med 2011;365:32–43.

24. Sackner-Bernstein JD, Kowalski M, Fox M, et al. Short-term risk of death after treatment with nesiritide for decompensated heart failure: a pooled analysis of randomized controlled trials. JAMA 2005;293: 1900–5.

A Review of Phase II Acute Heart Failure Syndromes Clinical Trials

Peter S. Pang, MD[a,b],*, Mihai Gheorghiade, MD[b]

KEYWORDS

• Acute heart failure • Clinical trials • Phase 2

More than 10 years have passed since the first large-scale clinical trials for acute heart failure syndromes (AHFS) were initially designed and then conducted. To date, every trial has disappointed, either failing in terms of efficacy or raising safety concerns.[1–8] Yet the need in AHFS remains as the postdischarge rehospitalization and mortality rate has changed little over the past decade, reaching as high as 50% within 60 to 90 days.[9] Heart failure (HF) is the most common reason for rehospitalization and the most expensive hospital diagnosis for Medicare beneficiaries, a fact worth highlighting given the aging of the population.[10] With more than 1 million admissions per year in the United States, consuming more than $20 million each year in HF care,[11–14] there continues to be an unmet need for novel therapies in AHFS.[10]

Why have trials failed? Lack of efficacy or safety concerns regarding the drug itself is the easiest explanation. Yet the substantial preclinical and early clinical development work, combined with the knowledge gained from previous trials, suggests that a lack of efficacy or concern for safety does not fully explain the lack of success seen with AHFS clinical trials to date.

One of the most striking findings when reviewing trials is the gap between the positive signals seen in phase II and the results seen in phase III. The fact that each phase III study conducted to date in AHFS was preceded by multiple positive phase II studies requires inquiry: are the right questions being asked during phase II (and if the right question, is it studied appropriately) that, if explored thoroughly, would lead to improved outcomes in phase III? Although the explanation for this gap is multifactorial, the authors focus on several broad themes. The first theme is the dose; the drug may be efficacious, but the wrong dose was chosen. The second theme relates to our limited understanding of the pathophysiology of AHFS, which may have resulted in a right drug/wrong target scenario. An ancillary theme would be an efficacious drug, but the hypothesis and, thus, target chosen was incorrect.[15] In this scenario, the wrong target suggests the possibilities of the wrong patient population, significant unaccounted

Disclosures for Peter Pang: Within the last 5 years, Peter Pang is or has been *Consultant for* Astellas, Bayer, EKR Therapeutics, J & J, Medtronic, the Medicines Company, Otsuka, Palatin Technologies, PDL BioPharma, Pericor Therapeutics, SigmaTau, Solvay Pharmaceuticals, and Trevena. *Honoraria* from BiogenIdec, Corthera, Ikaria, and Nile Therapeutics. *Research support* from Abbott, Merck, and PDL BioPharma.
Disclosures for Mihai Gheorghiade: Abbott Labs; Astellas; Astra Zeneca; Bayer Schering Pharma AG; CorThera, Inc; Cytokinetics, Inc; DebioPharm SA; Errekappa Terapeutici (Milan, Italy); Glaxo Smith Kline; Johnson & Johnson; Medtronic; Merck; Novartis Pharma AG; Otsuka Pharmaceuticals; Pericor Therapeutics; Protein Design Laboratories; Sanofi Aventis; Sigma Tau; and Solvay Pharmaceuticals.
[a] Department of Emergency Medicine, Northwestern University Feinberg School of Medicine, 211 East Ontario Street, Suite 200, Chicago, IL 60611, USA
[b] Center for Cardiovascular Innovation, Department of Medicine, Northwestern University Feinberg School of Medicine, 645 North Michigan Avenue, Suite 1006, Chicago, IL 60611, USA
* Corresponding author. Center for Cardiovascular Innovation, 645 North Michigan Avenue, Suite 1006, Chicago, IL 60611.
E-mail address: ppang@northwestern.edu

Heart Failure Clin 7 (2011) 441–450
doi:10.1016/j.hfc.2011.06.002

for differences within the target population (eg, genetic variations to drug response, heterogeneity in the patient population), or timing of intervention that may have missed the therapeutic window.[16–19] Finally, operational issues, such as poor protocol adherence, lack of true standard therapy in both the placebo and the active arm, discrepancies in the use of evidence-based therapy, and geographic differences in systems of health care delivery are other issues.

By carefully reviewing phase II studies, there may be lessons learned to aid in future development programs. The authors recognize the bias inherent to hindsight. Given that a consensus review has already been published that outlines past lessons learned in AHFS clinical trials overall,[20] the authors focus on lessons learned as they relate to phase II studies.

HETEROGENEITY: PATIENTS AND PATHOPHYSIOLOGY

The heterogeneity of the AHFS patient population has been well established, ranging from advanced HF with severely reduced systolic function to hypertensive emergencies and preserved systolic function, with a substantial variety in between.[20] Although patients with AHFS may be universally identified by the presence of signs and symptoms of HF at the time of presentation,[21] there is also a wide variety of pathophysiologic mechanisms that may contribute to each AHFS presentation.

What has become increasingly evident is that attempts to target all patients with AHFS with novel therapies has disappointed. A more common paradigm with recent trials has been to focus on subpopulations within the overall AHFS population, for example, patients with AHFS and hypertension. A comprehensive understanding of which patients will have the greatest (and safest) response is a key goal in phase II studies.

PURPOSE OF PHASE II TRIALS

The primary purpose of phase II studies is to determine a drug's efficacy in the target population of interest while carefully monitoring safety. The risk/benefit profile would ideally be understood to a sufficient degree to decide whether or not to proceed onto pivotal phase III trials.

Several other goals of phase II are as follows:

1. Determine the best dose to bring forward into phase III
2. Identify within the target population which subpopulation may have a better response
3. Evaluate the potential endpoints for phase III.

Given this broad framework, the authors now review phase II trials in AHFS to consider potential lessons learned to apply to future studies. Only phase II programs where phase III results have already been published are reviewed.

PHASE II TRIALS IN AHFS: TOLVAPTAN

The Acute and Chronic Therapeutic Impact of a Vasopressin Antagonist in Congestive Heart Failure (ACTIV in CHF) trial was the primary phase II study whose results drove the design of the pivotal phase III study, Efficacy of Vasopressin antagonism in Heart Failure Outcome Study with Tolvaptan (EVEREST). In patients with reduced ejection fraction (EF) hospitalized for worsening HF with signs of clinical congestion, ACTIV-CHF had 2 primary endpoints, one for the in-hospital phase (body weight reduction at 24 hours after randomization) and the other for the chronic phase or 60 days postdischarge (reduction of worsening CHF: death, rehospitalization, or unscheduled visits for HF).

ACTIV-CHF enrolled 319 patients in a 1:1:1:1 design (placebo, 30 mg, 60 mg, 90 mg). Of note, only a 3-fold difference in dose was tested. A statistically significant decrease in body weight was observed with all doses; however, the greatest decrease was with the 30-mg dose at 24 hours and the 60-mg dose by the time of discharge. Improvements in patient reported global status, as well as improvements in serum sodium were all observed. Positive trends as well as statistically significant improvement in 60-day mortality was seen overall and also in specific subgroups: hyponatremia, increased blood urea nitrogen, and congestion.

Based primarily on changes in body weight and improvement in serum sodium, the phase III study was developed. EVEREST was 3 trials in 1; 2 short-term trials designed to evaluate the effects of tolvaptan and signs/symptoms in the hospital and a combined long-term trial designed to evaluate tolvaptan's effects on morbidity and mortality.[2,3,22] Although tolvaptan demonstrated a modest but statistically significant difference in weight loss, no differences in global clinical status were seen.[2] In terms of long-term outcomes, no differences in cardiovascular mortality or HF hospitalization were observed.[3]

Mechanistic Understanding

Tolvaptan is an oral vasopressin 2 receptor antagonist designed to treat congestion through hypotonic fluid removal, which subsequently corrects hyponatremia. By its aquaretic mechanism, tolvaptan was hypothesized to improve hemodynamics.

However, at the time of the phase III trial design, a hemodynamic study had not yet been performed, although the Effect of Tolvaptan on hemodynamic Parameters in Subjects with Heart Failure (ECLIPSE) trial was later conducted, which demonstrated a modest hemodynamic benefit.[23] This lack of substantial benefit may have been affected by a vasopressin-2 receptor-only blocking effect, leaving V1 (vascular smooth muscle) receptors available for vasoconstriction, as well as potential adverse effects on the heart (LV hypertrophy/remodeling), cancelling out any beneficial hemodynamic effects.[24]

In retrospect, a better understanding of the physiology of fluid removal by tolvaptan may have been important. By its mechanism of action, tolvaptan does not eliminate sodium; yet, diuretic dosing was decreased during the trial. Because of its aquaretic effect, tolvaptan may increase intravascular volume by increasing intravascular osmolarity through free water excretion.

Choice of Endpoint

Endpoints for clinical trials encompass both scientific as well as regulatory concerns. Body weight was chosen as a primary target for tolvaptan development. It is a commonly used surrogate for overall volume status, with patients instructed to monitor daily weight because changes often result in medication adjustment.[13] Body weight is viewed as a marker of congestion, a known pathophysiologic target in AHFS.[25] However, scientific evidence and rationale support divergent perspectives on the importance of body weight, highlighting the lack of clearly established pathophysiologic targets and universally agreed upon endpoints in AHFS.

Dose

ACTIV-CHF tested only a 3-fold difference in dose with single-day dosing. Although pharmacokinetic studies demonstrated a sustained effect, the pharmacodynamic effects may have required dose titration or twice-a-day dosing. A retrospective analysis from EVEREST suggests that additional dosing may have yielded additional dyspnea improvement.[17]

Study Design

With a 48-hour enrollment window after admission, patients received significant therapeutic intervention for congestion before randomization, which may have blunted the potential symptom benefits of tolvaptan.[16,17] Post hoc analysis has demonstrated greater symptom improvement with earlier randomization.[17]

Overall, body weight decreased and serum sodium improved in ACTIV-CHF; however, no change in outcomes was seen, with a nonsignificant trend toward improvement in signs and symptoms during hospitalization.

PHASE II TRIALS IN AHFS: TEZOSENTAN

Tezosentan is a dual endothelin receptor antagonist designed to antagonize the deleterious effects of the endothelin neurohormone. Endothelins are peptide molecules with similar, but more potent, actions as angiotensin-II. Endothelins have been shown to be a strong prognostic marker for mortality and promote pathophysiologic processes in HF, such as vasoconstriction, proarrhythmogenesis, and further activation of neurohormones.[26–28] After an extensive phase II development program, the phase III pivotal Value of Endothelin Receptor Inhibition with Tezosentan in Acute heart failure Study (VERITAS) was designed to test whether parenteral tezosentan would improve symptoms and outcomes in addition to standard therapy versus standard therapy alone in patients with AHFS.

Prior to VERITAS, tezosentan was extensively studied in 4 phase II studies, known as the Randomized Intravenous Tezosentan Study (RITZ) trials (**Table 1**).[26,27,29] Because a complete overview of tezosentan development is beyond the scope of this article, the authors focus on 2 of the RITZ trials.

RITZ-1 tested whether a 24-hour infusion of 25 mg/h of tezosentan improved patients' self-assessed dyspnea at 24 hours after the start of infusion. No significant improvement in dyspnea was seen in 669 patients hospitalized for AHFS requiring intravenous (IV) therapy.

RITZ-2 demonstrated a significant and safe hemodynamic benefit with 6 hours of treatment with 50 and 100 mg of tezosentan, increasing the cardiac index and lowering the pulmonary capillary wedge pressure (PCWP) significantly versus placebo plus standard therapy. In addition, substantial dyspnea improvements were seen along with trends toward reduction in mortality and worsening HF. These dyspnea improvements were in contrast to the RITZ-1 findings.

An invasive hemodynamic dose-finding study was also conducted to determine the optimal efficacy/adverse effect dose.[30] Dosages were explored from 0.2 mg/h to 25 mg/h, a 500-fold difference when compared with the 100-mg/h dosage. Similar efficacy was seen with the 5-mg/h dosage as the 25-mg/h dosage when compared with the 50-mg/h dosage, with the 1-mg/h dosage having nearly the same hemodynamic effect as the 5-mg/h dosage. In addition, the effect of

Table 1
RITZ clinical development program

		Study Design	Primary Endpoint
RITZ-1[1] *A study to investigate the efficacy and safety of tezosentan in reducing symptoms in patients with acute decompensated HF*	n = 666	Multicenter, double blind, placebo controlled, RCT	Change in dyspnea at 24 h
RITZ-2[2] *Hemodynamic and clinical effects of tezosentan, an intravenous dual endothelin receptor antagonist, in patients hospitalized for acute decompensated HF*	n = 292	Multicenter, double blind, placebo controlled, RCT	Mean change in cardiac index from baseline to 6 h
RITZ-4[3] *Tezosentan in patients with acute HF and ACS*	n = 200	Multicenter, double blind placebo controlled, RCT	Composite of death, worsening HF, recurrent ischemia, and recurrent or new MI within 72 h
RITZ-5[4] *Randomized intravenous tezosentan for the treatment of pulmonary edema*	n = 84	Multicenter, double blind, placebo controlled, RCT	Change in oxygen saturation from baseline to 1 h

Abbreviation: RCT, randomized controlled trial.
Data from Refs.[29,33,52,53]

tezosentan on brain-type natriuretic peptide (BNP) levels was also measured, with significant differences in all treatment doses when compared with placebo.

Despite a robust phase II program with favorable signals, the phase III VERITAS program failed to meet its coprimary endpoint: sustained improvement in dyspnea at 24 hours and reduction in death or worsening HF at 7 days.[4]

Choice of Endpoint and Study Design

VERITAS demonstrated a rapid and sustained improvement in dyspnea in both the placebo and treatment arms.[4] This finding may reflect a limited ability to accurately and reliably measure dyspnea in AHFS.[16] Another possibility is that the rapid improvement in dyspnea by conventional therapy highlights the difficulty of targeting this endpoint.[4,16,18] The substantial improvement in the placebo (ie, standard therapy) arm seen in Vasodilation in the Management of Acute Congestive Heart Failure, EVEREST, VERITAS, and the URGENT-Dyspnea study demonstrates the efficacy of standard therapy.[2–4,8,18] Although the VERITAS window of enrollment (24 hours) was

one of the shortest for a large-scale trial to date, this may still be too late to capture dyspnea when it is most severe.[18] However, this degree of improvement has recently been challenged by results from the relaxin and rolofylline development programs, which demonstrate that requiring elevated BNP for inclusion criteria shows a significantly less proportion of patients with early dyspnea improvement.[31,32] Elevated BNP was not a mandatory requirement in VERITAS.

Interestingly, significant hemodynamic improvements seen in phase II did not result in dyspnea improvement versus standard therapy alone. This finding raises the question of the relationship between abnormal hemodynamics and the sensation of dyspnea and whether improvement in hemodynamics is a complete pathophysiologic explanation for improved dyspnea. Another potential explanation for the discord between RITZ-1 and 2 dyspnea results may have been caused by the bias introduced by invasive hemodynamic monitoring.[33]

Overall, the RITZ trials highlight a robust clinical development program, with careful attention to symptoms, invasive hemodynamics given the hemodynamic effects of tezosentan, adequate dose-finding, as well as a study in high-risk patients (eg, acute coronary syndromes [ACS] and AHFS).

PHASE II TRIALS IN AHFS: LEVOSIMENDAN

Levosimendan acts by 2 primary mechanisms: a calcium sensitizer to improve myocardial performance and as a vasodilator via actions on potassium ATP channels:[34,35] in effect, an inotropic-lusitropic vasodilator. Importantly, prior studies have shown that levosimendan improves cardiac performance without increasing myocardial oxygen demand.

The early levosimendan clinical development studies are summarized in **Table 2**. Two dose-finding studies were performed, one as dose ranging and the other as dose escalation, with a 12-fold difference in the loading dose and a 10-fold difference in the continuous infusion dose.[35,36] Clear dose-dependent invasive hemodynamic benefits were noted: increased cardiac index and a decrease in PCWP, without an increase in dysrhythmias.[35–37]

The Levosimendan Infusion versus Dobutamine in severe low output HF (LIDO) trial enrolled patients with a clinical need for a pulmonary artery line and IV inotropic support, with an EF less than 35%, a confidence interval (CI) less than 2.5 L/m²/min, and a mean PCWP greater than 15 mm Hg. The primary endpoint was hemodynamic improvement after 24 hours of continuous infusion as defined by a CI greater than or equal to 30% more than the baseline and PCWP less than or equal to 25% ($\geq$4 mm Hg) lower than the baseline, and not needing rescue therapy with other IV positive inotropic agents or vasodilators.[37] Levosimendan, when compared with dobutamine, demonstrated a statistically significant greater proportion of patients who met the primary endpoint. In addition, by time-to-event analysis, a greater number of patients in the levosimendan arm remained event free, defined by a combined risk of death or worsening HF at 31 days.[37]

Levosimendan was also studied in patients after myocardial infarction (MI) in The Randomized Study on Safety and Effectiveness of Levosimendan in Patients with Left Ventricular Failure after Acute Myocardial Infarct (RUSSLAN) trial.[38] In this parallel group study (5 arms), with the exception of the highest dose, there was no more ischemia or clinically relevant hypotension when compared with placebo. In addition, the secondary endpoint of worsening death at 14 days was less in the levosimendan arms.

Table 2
Levosimendan clinical development program

Dose Escalation[1] *Acute hemodynamic and clinical effects of levosimendan in patients with severe HF*	n = 146	Multicenter, double blind, placebo controlled, RCT	Proportion of patients with an increase in SV or a decrease in PCWP of 25% at 6 h
Dose Ranging[2] *Hemodynamic and neurohumoral effects of continuous infusion of levosimendan in patients with congestive HF*	n = 151	Multicenter, double blind, placebo controlled, parallel group, RCT	Responders analysis based on a combination of prespecified changes in CO, PCWP, and SV
LIDO[3] *Efficacy and safety of intravenous levosimendan compared with dobutamine in severe low-output HF (the LIDO study)*	n = 203	Multicenter, double blind, placebo controlled, parallel group, RCT	Proportion of patients with hemodynamic improvement (defined as an increase of 30% or more in CO and a decrease of 25% or more in pulmonary-capillary wedge pressure) at 24 h
RUSSLAN[4] *Safety and efficacy of a novel calcium sensitizer, levosimendan, in patients with left ventricular failure caused by an acute MI*	n = 504	Multicenter, double blind, placebo controlled, RCT	Hypotension or myocardial ischemia of clinical significance adjudicated by an independent safety committee

Abbreviations: CO, cardiac output; RCT, randomized controlled trial; SV, stroke volume.
Data from Refs.[35–38]

The CAlcium Sensitizer or Inotrope or NOne in low output heart failure (CASINO) trial, which has not yet been published, was a randomized, double-blind, placebo-controlled, parallel group trial of levosimendan versus dobutamine versus placebo that was halted after 277 patients were enrolled, which was less than half of the 600 patient planned enrollment. A statistically significant reduction in death at the 1-month and 6-month follow-up was noted, leading investigators to halt the study.[39]

These results influenced the design of the REVIVE trials (Randomized Evaluations of Levosimendan). REVIVE I (levosimendan vs placebo) was designed as a pilot study to evaluate a novel composite endpoint for AHFS trials, highlighting the importance of both early and sustained improvements in symptoms without worsening HF or other morbid/mortal events.[40] Based on the positive pilot results, the endpoint was further refined to demonstrate an even earlier benefit (at 6 hours vs 24 hours) as well as a more stringent definition of worsening HF (rescue diuretics after 72 hours vs rescue diuretics at any time).

REVIVE-2 demonstrated a statistically significant improvement in the composite endpoint compared with placebo. In addition, significant improvements in secondary endpoints, such as reduction in BNP at 24 hours, improved patient global assessment at 6 hours, as well as dyspnea assessments at 6 hours, all favored levosimendan. In addition, hospital length of stay significantly favored levosimendan versus placebo.[41]

However, there was a trend toward greater adverse events (hypotension, ventricular tachycardia, atrial fibrillation) as well as serious adverse events (mortality) in the patients treated with levosimendan.[41,42] Based on the totality of the development program, the pivotal phase III trial, Survival of Patients With Acute Heart Failure in Need of Intravenous Inotropic Support (SURVIVE) (levosimendan vs dobutamine for patients with acute decompensated HF) was designed.

SURVIVE was a mortality trial of levosimendan versus dobutamine in patients with reduced EF less than 35%, hospitalized for AHFS, and a clinical need for inotropic support.[5] Despite the trends toward improvement seen in the majority of the phase II studies, but importantly not in the REVIVE studies, SURVIVE failed to achieve the primary endpoint of less 180-day all-cause mortality when compared with dobutamine.[5]

Mechanistic Understanding and Study Design

During the design of the REVIVE and SURVIVE trials, experience with levosimendan was considerable in several European countries. Although clinicians observed hypotension with bolus dosing, the bolus was continued in the design of SURVIVE. Although levosimendan was developed as an inotrope, its vasodilatory properties were identified early given its potassium ATP channel activity. Whether this hypotension may have significantly affected coronary perfusion leading to worse events has been proposed as one potential mechanism. In hindsight, it is possible that a potential mismatch occurred in the chosen target population, given its inodilatory effects.

The timing of enrollment in SURVIVE was also late: up to 48 hours after admission. Potentially, less hemodynamic benefit may have been realized given the introduction of earlier upstream therapies.

PHASE II TRIALS IN AHFS: ROLOFYLLINE

Worsening renal function, defined as a change in serum creatinine (Cr) of 0.3 or greater, is a significant predictor of morbidity and mortality in patients with AHFS.[43–45] These findings led to the hypothesis that prevention of worsening renal function leads to improved outcomes in patients with AHFS. Rolofylline is an adenosine-1 receptor antagonist developed to protect the kidney from worsening renal function during decompensated HF.[46] Its primary mechanism of action is twofold: (1) enhance diuresis by inhibition of sodium reabsorption in the proximal tubule and (2) maintain glomerular filtration rate (GFR) by blocking adenosine mediated vasoconstriction of the afferent arteriole.[47]

Phase II development of rolofylline was tested in 3 separate studies: CKI-201, 202, and 203.[48,49]

CKI-201 enrolled 159 patients with a mean Cr of 45 mL/min in a dose-ranging study, with an approximate 25-fold difference between the lowest dosage (2.5 mg and 60.0 mg) infused for 2 hours over 3 days. IV loop diuretics were required before the initial dose, held for the first 6 hours after the start of infusion, and were then dosed per the investigators discretion 6 hours after the start of the infusion. At 6 hours, approximately 250 mL of greater urine output was seen with the 30-mg dose. However, less of a diuretic response was seen with the 60-mg dose. In terms of diuretic dosing, the cumulative total at 7 days was greatest with the placebo, with similar cumulative dosing with the 15-mg and 30-mg dose, slightly higher with the 2.5-mg dose, and slightly lower with the 60-mg dose.[48]

CKI-202 tested the effects of rolofylline in diuretic-resistant patients with the New York Heart

Association (NYHA) class III/IV HF, with acute decompensation and severe renal impairment (mean creatine clearance [CrCl] 34). A substantial difference in the primary endpoint, urine output, was seen with rolofylline at all doses, with the greatest effect seen within the first 3 hours after dosing. Again, a U-shaped dose response was seen early, with a 30-mg dose yielding greater urine output than the 60-mg dose. In terms of the secondary endpoint, change in CrCl from the baseline, the 30-mg dose demonstrated a substantial improvement compared with all other doses, with the 60-mg dose showing worse CrCl when compared with placebo by 24 hours.

CKI-203 tested rolofylline in stable patients with HF with mild renal impairment in a randomized, 2-way crossover study (n = 32) with background furosemide therapy.[49] A persistent improvement in GFR was seen with rolofylline, exhibiting a pharmacodynamic effect beyond that attributable to its pharmacokinetic profile. Interestingly, however, the placebo arm also showed an improvement in GFR during therapy, albeit less substantial; however, GFR dropped to below the baseline after the washout period.

Benefits seen during early phase II studies led to the design of the PROTECT pilot study (A Study of the Selective A1 Adenosine Receptor Antagonist KW-3902 for Patients Hospitalized With Acute HF and Volume Overload to Assess Treatment Effect on Congestion and Renal Function). The PROTECT Pilot was designed to answer 3 primary objectives: final dose finding, appropriateness of the primary end point and sample size calculations, and safely, especially in regard to seizure prevention.[32] Importantly, the study was not powered to answer any specific hypothesis; instead the 301 patients enrolled were analyzed post hoc based on the endpoints chosen for the phase III study. This study had a trichotomous endpoint: (1) *treatment success* on days 2 and 3, which was defined as dyspnea reported by the patient as moderately or markedly better compared with the study start, and not a treatment failure; (2) *treatment failure,* which includes any 1 of the following criteria: death or readmission for HF through day 7, worsening symptoms or signs of HF, and persistent renal impairment (serum creatinine increases $\geq$0.3 mg/dL at day 7 and confirmed at day 14); and (3) *patient unchanged*: neither treatment success nor treatment failure.[32]

Results from the PROTECT pilot demonstrated a larger proportion of patients with treatment success and less failure in the 30-mg dose group compared with placebo. Additionally, an improvement in serum creatinine was seen at day 14, which trended toward significance when compared with worsening renal function seen in the other dose groups, with the worst renal function at day 14 in the placebo arm.[32] Trends toward less death and rehospitalization were also seen with the 30-mg dose.

The combination of phase II data along with the PROTECT pilot study led to the phase III PROTECT study, which ultimately failed to achieve its primary endpoint, based on a slightly modified trichotomous endpoint based on the pilot results.[50,51] In addition, the secondary endpoints (time to death or rehospitalization at 60 days or the proportion of patients with persistent renal impairment at day 7 and day 14) were also not achieved.[51]

MECHANISTIC UNDERSTANDING AND STUDY DESIGN

Given the mechanistic hypothesis that rolofylline protects or preserves renal function compared with standard therapy, hindsight suggests that in spite of a clear trend, an adequately powered study to test this hypothesis should have been performed. However, this may not have changed the outcome because the proportion of patients with persistent renal impairment at days 7 and 14, (11% in the placebo arm) was less than anticipated. It has been suggested that the education of investigators regarding the cardiorenal syndrome and the potential deleterious effects of loop diuretic therapy may have contributed.

Finally, although the 30-mg dose was chosen based on adverse events (eg, safety), the U-shaped dose response was not adequately explained. In other words, why the 60-mg dose had less diuretic effect, or in 1 the phase II study show worsening in CrCl compared with placebo, may have been a signal to investigate further.

SUMMARY

A significant need exists for new therapies to treat AHFS given the high postdischarge mortality and rehospitalization rate. Despite the largely disappointing results of clinical trials to date, much has been learned. Phase II trials have demonstrated scientific rigor and ingenuity. At the same time, in hindsight, there is an overall lack of consistency between trials and a failure to address what may have been pivotal questions unique to each development program before the launch of phase III. Although not specifically discussed, it is clear that multiple factors other than scientific ones are important for clinical development, such as business development, patent life, or regulatory concerns. Regardless, lack of success to date, combined with the tremendous unmet need, suggests that even greater methodological rigor before phase III may be an important strategy to consider in future development.

REFERENCES

1. Cuffe MS, Califf RM, Adams KF Jr, et al. Short-term intravenous milrinone for acute exacerbation of chronic heart failure: a randomized controlled trial. JAMA 2002;287:1541–7.

2. Gheorghiade M, Konstam MA, Burnett JC Jr, et al. Short-term clinical effects of tolvaptan, an oral vasopressin antagonist, in patients hospitalized for heart failure: the EVEREST Clinical Status Trials. JAMA 2007;297(12):1332–43.

3. Konstam MA, Gheorghiade M, Burnett JC Jr, et al. Effects of oral tolvaptan in patients hospitalized for worsening heart failure: the EVEREST Outcome Trial. JAMA 2007;297(12):1319–31.

4. McMurray JJ, Teerlink JR, Cotter G, et al. Effects of tezosentan on symptoms and clinical outcomes in patients with acute heart failure: the VERITAS Randomized Controlled Trials. JAMA 2007;298(17):2009–19.

5. Mebazaa A, Nieminen MS, Packer M, et al. Levosimendan vs dobutamine for patients with acute decompensated heart failure: the SURVIVE Randomized Trial. JAMA 2007;297(17):1883–91.

6. Sackner-Bernstein JD, Kowalski M, Fox M, et al. Short-term risk of death after treatment with nesiritide for decompensated heart failure: a pooled analysis of randomized controlled trials. JAMA 2005;293(15):1900–5.

7. Sackner-Bernstein JD, Skopicki HA, Aaronson KD. Risk of worsening renal function with nesiritide in patients with acutely decompensated heart failure. Circulation 2005;111(12):1487–91.

8. VMAC Investigators. Intravenous nesiritide vs nitroglycerin for treatment of decompensated congestive heart failure: a randomized controlled trial. JAMA 2002;287(12):1531–40.

9. Gheorghiade M, Abraham WT, Albert NM, et al. Systolic blood pressure at admission, clinical characteristics, and outcomes in patients hospitalized with acute heart failure. JAMA 2006;296(18):2217–26.

10. Jencks SF, Williams MV, Coleman EA. Rehospitalizations among patients in the Medicare fee-for-service program. N Engl J Med 2009;360(14):1418–28.

11. Dickstein K, Cohen-Solal A, Filippatos G, et al. ESC Guidelines for the diagnosis and treatment of acute and chronic heart failure 2008: the Task Force for the diagnosis and treatment of acute and chronic heart failure 2008 of the European Society of Cardiology. Developed in collaboration with the Heart Failure Association of the ESC (HFA) and endorsed by the European Society of Intensive Care Medicine (ESICM). Eur Heart J 2008;29(19):2388–442.

12. Fang J, Mensah GA, Croft JB, et al. Heart failure-related hospitalization in the U.S., 1979 to 2004. J Am Coll Cardiol 2008;52(6):428–34.

13. Hunt SA, Abraham WT, Chin MH, et al. 2009 focused update incorporated into the ACC/AHA 2005 Guidelines for the Diagnosis and Management of Heart Failure in Adults A Report of the American College of Cardiology Foundation/American Heart Association Task Force on Practice Guidelines Developed in Collaboration With the International Society for Heart and Lung Transplantation. J Am Coll Cardiol 2009;53(15):e1–90.

14. Lloyd-Jones D, Adams R, Carnethon M, et al. Heart disease and stroke statistics–2009 update: a report from the American Heart Association Statistics Committee and Stroke Statistics Subcommittee. Circulation 2009;119(3):480–6.

15. Yancy CW. Climbing the mountain of acute decompensated heart failure: the EVEREST Trials. JAMA 2007;297(12):1374–6.

16. Pang PS, Cleland JG, Teerlink JR, et al. A proposal to standardize dyspnoea measurement in clinical trials of acute heart failure syndromes: the need for a uniform approach. Eur Heart J 2008;29(6):816–24.

17. Pang PS, Konstam MA, Krasa HB, et al. Effects of tolvaptan on dyspnoea relief from the EVEREST trials. Eur Heart J 2009;30(18):2233–40.

18. Mebazaa A, Pang PS, Tavares M, et al. The impact of early standard therapy on dyspnoea in patients with acute heart failure: the URGENT-dyspnoea study. Eur Heart J 2009;31(7):832–41.

19. Blair JE, Zannad F, Konstam MA, et al. Continental differences in clinical characteristics, management, and outcomes in patients hospitalized with worsening heart failure results from the EVEREST (Efficacy of Vasopressin Antagonism in Heart Failure: Outcome Study with Tolvaptan) program. J Am Coll Cardiol 2008;52(20):1640–8.

20. Felker GM, Pang PS, Adams KF, et al. Clinical trials of pharmacological therapies in acute heart failure syndromes: lessons learned and directions forward. Circ Heart Fail 2010;3(2):314–25.

21. Gheorghiade M, Zannad F, Sopko G, et al. Acute heart failure syndromes: current state and framework for future research. Circulation 2005;112(25):3958–68.

22. Gheorghiade M, Gattis WA, Barbagelata A, et al. Rationale and study design for a multicenter, randomized, double-blind, placebo-controlled study of the effects of tolvaptan on the acute and chronic outcomes of patients hospitalized with worsening congestive heart failure. Am Heart J 2003;145(Suppl 2):S51–4.

23. Udelson JE, Orlandi C, Ouyang J, et al. Acute hemodynamic effects of tolvaptan, a vasopressin V2 receptor blocker, in patients with symptomatic heart

failure and systolic dysfunction: an international, multicenter, randomized, placebo-controlled trial. J Am Coll Cardiol 2008;52(19):1540–5.

24. Goldsmith SR, Gheorghiade M. Vasopressin antagonism in heart failure. J Am Coll Cardiol 2005;46: 1785–91.

25. Gheorghiade M, Filippatos G, De Luca L, et al. Congestion in acute heart failure syndromes: an essential target of evaluation and treatment. Am J Med 2006;119(12 Suppl 1):S3–10.

26. Teerlink JR. Overview of randomized clinical trials in acute heart failure syndromes. Am J Cardiol 2005; 96(6A):59G–67G.

27. Teerlink JR, McMurray JJ, Bourge RC, et al. Tezosentan in patients with acute heart failure: design of the Value of Endothelin Receptor Inhibition with Tezosentan in Acute heart failure Study (VERITAS). Am Heart J 2005;150(1):46–53.

28. Aronson D, Burger AJ. Neurohumoral activation and ventricular arrhythmias in patients with decompensated congestive heart failure: role of endothelin. Pacing Clin Electrophysiol 2003;26(3):703–10.

29. O'Connor CM, Gattis WA, Adams KF Jr, et al. Tezosentan in patients with acute heart failure and acute coronary syndromes: results of the Randomized Intravenous TeZosentan Study (RITZ-4). J Am Coll Cardiol 2003;41(9):1452–7.

30. Cotter G, Kaluski E, Stangl K, et al. The hemodynamic and neurohormonal effects of low doses of tezosentan (an endothelin A/B receptor antagonist) in patients with acute heart failure. Eur J Heart Fail 2004;6(5):601–9.

31. Teerlink JR, Metra M, Felker GM, et al. Relaxin for the treatment of patients with acute heart failure (Pre-RELAX-AHF): a multicentre, randomised, placebo-controlled, parallel-group, dose-finding phase IIb study. Lancet 2009;373(9673):1429–39.

32. Cotter G, Dittrich HC, Weatherley BD, et al. The PROTECT pilot study: a randomized, placebo-controlled, dose-finding study of the adenosine A1 receptor antagonist rolofylline in patients with acute heart failure and renal impairment. J Card Fail 2008; 14(8):631–40.

33. Teerlink JR. Dyspnea as an end point in clinical trials of therapies for acute decompensated heart failure. Am Heart J 2003;145(Suppl 2):S26–33.

34. Gheorghiade M, Teerlink JR, Mebazaa A. Pharmacology of new agents for acute heart failure syndromes. Am J Cardiol 2005;96(6A):68G–73G.

35. Slawsky MT, Colucci WS, Gottlieb SS, et al. Acute hemodynamic and clinical effects of levosimendan in patients with severe heart failure. Study Investigators. Circulation 2000;102(18):2222–7.

36. Nieminen MS, Akkila J, Hasenfuss G, et al. Hemodynamic and neurohumoral effects of continuous infusion of levosimendan in patients with congestive heart failure. J Am Coll Cardiol 2000;36(6):1903–12.

37. Follath F, Cleland JG, Just H, et al. Efficacy and safety of intravenous levosimendan compared with dobutamine in severe low-output heart failure (the LIDO study): a randomised double-blind trial. Lancet 2002;360(9328):196–202.

38. Moiseyev VS, Poder P, Andrejevs N, et al. Safety and efficacy of a novel calcium sensitizer, levosimendan, in patients with left ventricular failure due to an acute myocardial infarction. A randomized, placebo-controlled, double-blind study (RUSSLAN). Eur Heart J 2002;23(18):1422–32.

39. Zairis MN, Apostolatos C, Anastasiadis P, et al. 835-6 The effect of a calcium sensitizer or an inotrope or none in chronic low output decompensated heart failure: results from the calcium sensitizer or inotrope or none in low output heart failure study (CASINO). J Am Coll Cardiol 2004;43(5 Suppl 1):A206–7.

40. Packer M, Colucci WS, Fisher L. Development of a comprehensive new endpoint for the evaluation of new treatments for acute decompensated heart failure: results with levosimendan in the REVIVE-1 study [abstract]. J Card Fail 2003;9:S61.

41. Packer M. REVIVE II: Multicenter placebo-controlled trial of levosimendan on clinical status in acutely decompensated heart failure [abstract]. Paper presented at: American Heart Association Scientific Sessions 2005 Late Breaking Clinical Trials II. Dallas, November 13–16, 2005.

42. Packer M. The Randomized multicenter EValuation of Intravenous leVosimendan Efficacy-2 (REVIVE-2) trial, Late-breaking Clinical Trials. Dallas (TX): American Heart Association, Annual Scientific Session; 2005. p. 13–6.

43. Gottlieb SS, Abraham W, Butler J, et al. The prognostic importance of different definitions of worsening renal function in congestive heart failure. J Card Fail 2002;8(3):136–41.

44. Smith GL, Lichtman JH, Bracken MB, et al. Renal impairment and outcomes in heart failure: systematic review and meta-analysis. J Am Coll Cardiol 2006;47(10):1987–96.

45. Smith GL, Vaccarino V, Kosiborod M, et al. Worsening renal function: what is a clinically meaningful change in creatinine during hospitalization with heart failure? J Card Fail 2003;9(1):13–25.

46. Gottlieb SS, Brater DC, Thomas I, et al. BG9719 (CVT-124), an A1 adenosine receptor antagonist, protects against the decline in renal function observed with diuretic therapy. Circulation 2002;105(11):1348–53.

47. Gottlieb SS, Skettino SL, Wolff A, et al. Effects of BG9719 (CVT-124), an A1-adenosine receptor antagonist, and furosemide on glomerular filtration rate and natriuresis in patients with congestive heart failure. J Am Coll Cardiol 2000;35(1):56–9.

48. Givertz MM, Massie BM, Fields TK, et al. The effects of KW-3902, an adenosine A1-receptor antagonist, on diuresis and renal function in patients with acute

decompensated heart failure and renal impairment or diuretic resistance. J Am Coll Cardiol 2007; 50(16):1551–60.

49. Dittrich HC, Gupta DK, Hack TC, et al. The effect of KW-3902, an adenosine A1 receptor antagonist, on renal function and renal plasma flow in ambulatory patients with heart failure and renal impairment. J Card Fail 2007;13(8):609–17.

50. Weatherley BD, Cotter G, Dittrich HC, et al. Design and rationale of the PROTECT study: a placebo-controlled randomized study of the selective A1 adenosine receptor antagonist rolofylline for patients hospitalized with acute decompensated heart failure and volume overload to assess treatment effect on congestion and renal function. J Card Fail 2010;16(1):25–35.

51. Massie BM, O'Connor CM, Metra M, et al. Rolofylline, an adenosine A1-receptor antagonist, in acute heart failure. N Engl J Med 2010;363(15): 1419–28.

52. Torre-Amione G, Young JB, Colucci WS, et al. Hemodynamic and clinical effects of tezosentan, an intravenous dual endothelin receptor antagonist, in patients hospitalized for acute decompensated heart failure. J Am Coll Cardiol 2003;42(1):140–7.

53. Kaluski E, Kobrin I, Zimlichman R, et al. RITZ-5: randomized intravenous TeZosentan (an endothelin-A/B antagonist) for the treatment of pulmonary edema: a prospective, multicenter, double-blind, placebo-controlled study. J Am Coll Cardiol 2003; 41(2):204–10.

Lessons Learned from Clinical Trials in Acute Heart Failure: Phase 3 Drug Trials

Christopher M. O'Connor, MD[a],*, Mona Fiuzat, PharmD[b]

KEYWORDS

• Acute heart failure • Phase 3 clinical trials • Endpoints
• Efficacy • Safety

Phase 3 clinical trials in acute heart failure (AHF) are conducted to allow safety and efficacy data to be collected for the evaluation of treatment strategies, including drugs, devices, diagnostics, or nonpharmacological interventions. Phase 3 trials occur after there has been satisfactory information gathered on animal studies and early phase studies, such that the safety, pharmacokinetic, and dosing profiles have been adequately ascertained. The phase 3 study is then designed to test the efficacy and safety of the intervention in a larger sample size. There are several important features regarding the conduct of phase 3 clinical trials in AHF. This article describes in detail these important aspects of conducting phase 3 clinical trials in an AHF population.

STUDY DESIGN

In the planning of an AHF trial, one of the most important determinants of the scope of the trial is the question being asked. Stating the question clearly and in advance allows the investigative team to properly design the study. Each clinical trial has a primary question, which should be clearly defined in advance and stated as such in the protocol. Numerous secondary questions are often asked, and these should be put in descending order of importance. Primary and secondary questions should be important and relevant to the field of acute decompensated heart failure. As always, patient safety and well being should be considered in evaluating the importance of the questions asked.

The key to developing the question is to have a clear understanding of the type of intervention, including the dose, frequency, and duration of administration of therapy, whether it is a drug, device, or behavioral intervention. In acute decompensated heart failure trials, aspects such as timing of initiation, duration of the intervention, logistics of blinding, and location of study patients pose particular challenges in the design of phase 3 studies. For example, it is highly unlikely to expect that a therapy could be administered routinely within 1 hour of presentation to the emergency room, given the challenges in ascertaining the diagnosis of the patient, unlike a patient with ST segment elevation myocardial infarction (STEMI) or a patient in cardiogenic shock.

One of the most important aspects of phase 3 studies in AHF is the study population. Defining the population in advance and stating very clearly the inclusion and exclusion criteria are important as one draws conclusions at the end of a trial. This aspect also impacts recruitment. As often seen, the study population is truly a subset of the general population of the disease state being studied. How this differs from registries is important in the generalizability of results. Careful characterization of the study population is essential for the proper interpretation of the trial. In general, subjects who have the potential to benefit from the intervention are the candidates for participation in the study. If the mechanism of action of the intervention is precisely known, then a more homogenous population can be studied. For

[a] Division of Cardiology, Duke University Medical Center, DUMC 3356, Durham, NC 27710, USA
[b] Duke University Medical Center, 2400 Pratt Street, Room 8011, Durham, NC 27710, USA
* Corresponding author.
E-mail address: Oconn002@mc.duke.edu

Heart Failure Clin 7 (2011) 451–456
doi:10.1016/j.hfc.2011.06.013

example, patients with acute decompensated heart failure who have a wide QRS interval may be candidates for a randomized controlled study of biventricular pacing versus usual care. However, if the mechanism of action of the intervention is not known or multifactorial in its potential for benefit, a broader, more heterogeneous population may participate in the study. The degree of homogeneity or heterogeneity may evolve over time. As the underlying disease process is better understood, more targeted interventions to subpopulations may be more prudent for determining a greater response.

Additionally, the safety profile is important in determining the patient population of a study. Subjects such as pregnant women or the very elderly (ie, >age 90) may be excluded from studies. However, the broader the population, the more one can generalize the results. Recently, it has been very important to identify and enhance the enrollment of patients of special populations such as the elderly, women, and minorities, and from different geographic regions, enhancing one's ability to draw conclusions in these subgroups.

RANDOMIZATION AND BLINDING

Fundamental to phase 3 clinical trials in AHF is randomization. This ensures that patients are equally likely to be assigned to either the intervention or the control group. The advantages of randomization are multifactorial.

First, it removes potential bias in the allocation of patients to either group. Second, it provides comparable groups in the intervention and control group. Third, it allows to the validity of statistical testing. When randomization is not used, assumptions regarding the comparability of the groups and the types of statistical tests in models must be made, which increase the difficulty of interpretation. Randomization can be done with several methods. Fixed allocated randomization allows an equal allocation of the probability of receiving the intervention or the control, which is not altered as the study is conducted. Some advocate unequal allocation such as 2:1 or 3:2 randomization interventions in the control. Simple randomization is usually conducted by development of a random number generated by algorithm, and allocating patients to 1 treatment group or the other. Block randomization technique is used to avoid large imbalances in the number of patients assigned to a group. Patients have equal probability to treatment assignment, and are allocated in blocks of even size such as 6 or 8. Stratified randomization is another way to prevent imbalance. These variables are factors that correlate with a subject response or outcome in an attempt to balance randomization within each stratum, to prevent an imbalanced response at the end of the trial. There are also methods of adaptive randomization; that is, to adjust the randomization based on information as the trial is ongoing. In general, large phase 3 studies generally use block randomization. Stratified randomization is generally not necessary in trials in which there are over several thousand patients enrolled, because the balance of randomization is usually guaranteed among the important prognostic variables. For smaller studies, randomization could be blocked or stratified based on a few important factors. Adaptive randomization strategies are also used in smaller-sized studies.

In phase 3 AHF trials, blinding is also an important component of the study design. To avoid potential issues of bias during data collection assessments, particularly subjective assessments such as dyspnea or physician global assessment, a double-blind design should be instituted. In studies where such a design is not possible, a single-blind approach should be used with independent core laboratories for primary and secondary endpoints.

SAMPLE SIZE

Sample sizes should have sufficient statistical power to detect differences between groups; therefore, issues regarding sample size calculations are extremely important. One of the most important challenges is the adjustment of sample size to compensate for noncompliance to intervention and low event rates. Patients in the active treatment group who do not comply are often termed dropouts. Similarly, a controlled patient who begins to take active therapy is considered a drop-in. Therefore, attention must be made with estimates of the potential dropout rate. A simple way to estimate this is to multiply the sample size by $(1-R^2)$. For example, a dropout rate of 25% would increase the sample size by greater than 75%. Sample sizes for testing equivalency of interventions are even more difficult. These often require sample sizes of much greater than those of superiority trials, and can be significantly influenced by drop-in and dropout rates.

CLINICALLY RELEVANT ENDPOINTS IN AHF TRIALS

Response variables are the outcomes being measured during the course of the trial, and define and answer the questions being asked. In general, a single response variable should be identified to answer the primary question by the investigator. Occasionally, more than 1 response variable is a primary concern and thus, coprimary endpoints are defined. However, the probability of getting a significant result by chance alone is increased. In addition, when there are several response variables that are considered the coprimary endpoints, inconsistent results appear, and interpretation may become difficult. As in all major cardiovascular trials, combining events to make a combined endpoint has been useful. In acute decompensated heart failure, the combination of morbidity and mortality as an intermediate term outcome such as 30 days or 60 days has been used. The combined endpoint should be capable of meaningful interpretation, and only 1 event per subject should be counted. Additionally, the primary response variable, whether it is a single variable or composite variable, needs to be assessed in all subjects. Large amounts of missing variables of the primary endpoint can make interpretation of the results quite difficult. Third, it is important that response variables are capable of unbiased assessment. Double-blind studies have the advantage of protecting against this, but independent adjudication committees have become a standard mechanism in assuring standardization and blinded assessments. It is important to remember that in all acute decompensated heart failure trials of phase 3 status, there is a compromise between the ideal and practical issues of selection and measurement of the primary response variable. Attempting to get a response variable that can be reliably assessed and yet provide an answer to the primary question is a difficult balance. However, if such a response cannot be found, the intent to conduct the trial should be reevaluated.

In 2010, response variables of the highest significance in phase 3 studies included dyspnea relief, patient global assessment, and in-hospital clinical comorbid events such as in-hospital worsening heart failure, cardiovascular events, or death at 30 and 60 days. Mortality, total hospitalizations, cardiovascular hospitalizations, heart failure hospitalizations, and total days alive free of hospitalization in a time period represent the most robust clinical endpoints in ADHF trials. Additionally, quality-of-life measures such as the Kansas City Cardiomyopathy Questionnaire (KCCQ) and the Minnesota Living with Heart Failure Questionnaire (MLHFQ) would also be of importance at these intermediate time points.

SAFETY MEASUREMENTS IN AHF TRIALS

Additional aspects that can be addressed through the phase 3 clinical trial include the profile of adverse events. The description of what adverse reactions may occur to therapeutic interventions and their severity may be unpredictable until large numbers of patients are studied, such as in phase 3 studies. Having a database of over 1000 patients in a clinical study allows one to observe and describe rare but serious toxicities that have potentially not been described previously in smaller studies. Reaching statistical significance is often not possible with the small numbers. Clinically meaningful differences are one of the many positive aspects of doing the large-scale phase 3 studies.

While it is not necessarily for the primary intent of the study, additional information regarding the natural history of the disease state can be ascertained in a phase 3 trial. Particularly in large-scale studies, the demographics and simplified entry criteria may begin to mirror what a registry of patients appears to look like. For example, in the Acute Study of Clinical Effectiveness of Nesiritide in Decompensated Heart Failure (ASCEND-HF) trial of over 7000 patients, the demographics look very similar to the previously described The Organized Program to Initiate Lifesaving Treatment in Hospitalized Patients with Heart Failure (OPTIMIZE) and The Acute Decompensated Heart Failure National Registry (ADHERE) clinical registries of acute decompensated heart failure patients.[1,2] Providing additional information regarding the demographics, the clinical care provided, and event rates allow one to advance the field with important new knowledge.

Ancillary questions are often extremely important in phase 3 clinical trials. These questions are secondary questions set up with specific sample sizes and response variables, but can often provide valuable information in the study population.

LESSONS LEARNED FROM PHASE 3 TRIALS IN AHF

The history of phase 3 trials in acute decompensated heart failure can be examined through the analysis of the several major trials to date. The first 2 major phase 3 studies in AHF were the Vasodilation in the Management of Acute Congestive Heart Failure (V-MAC) and The Outcomes of a Prospective *Trial* of Intravenous Milrinone for Exacerbations of Chronic Heart Failure (OPTIME) trials.[3,4]

The OPTIME trial was a randomized controlled trial of intravenous milrinone in patients presenting with acute decompensated heart failure. This was the first established AHF trial with a sufficient number of patients enrolled (ie, adequate sample size and power to detect clinically meaningful differences). In the overall study, it was found that there was no difference between milrinone and placebo, with a primary endpoint of days alive out of the hospital at 60 days. Furthermore, there were an increased number of serious cardiovascular adverse events with milrinone, including hypotension and atrial and ventricular arrhythmias. The OPTIME trial highlighted a number of important issues:

Clinical outcome trials could be conducted in acute decompensated heart failure.

The patient population may respond differently based on heart failure etiology.

It is important to enroll a large number of patients.

There appeared to be a trend toward improvement of outcomes with a nonischemic etiology, and worse outcome with ischemic etiology. Finally, the trial showed that a relationship between hypotension, renal dysfunction, and worsening in-hospital heart failure is a theme that has to be examined carefully in drugs that have vasodilator components. In addition, there was an extraordinarily high event rate at 30 and 60 days in this AHF population, with a 20% rehospitalization and nearly 10% mortality rate, thus a combined rate of 30%. This provides an adequate target for conducting clinical outcome trials in AHF.

The V-MAC study randomized 489 patients to the novel vasodilator nesiritide versus placebo. The findings showed a statistically significant improvement in dyspnea with treatment. There also appeared to be an advantage in hemodynamics over nitroglycerin with respect to pulmonary capillary wedge pressure. The combined findings in this trial allowed for US Food and Drug Administration (FDA) approval of the drug. This was the first time a drug was approved for acute decompensated heart failure, beyond drugs that influence hemodynamics such as intravenous milrinone. In addition, using a clinically meaningful symptom such as dyspnea as an approvable and acceptable endpoint was an important first among the academic community, regulatory authorities, and the industry. The measurement of symptoms such as dyspnea or patient global assessment is challenging and has not been validated in the acute decompensated heart failure arena. Whether a Likert or visual analog scale is better is unclear, and blinding issues are extremely challenging. In the case of V-MAC, there was some concern that unmasking of the treatment could have occurred because of the change in hemodynamics, which could have influenced dyspnea assessments. Subsequently, the authors learned from V-MAC that the trial was not of sufficient size to comment on important safety parameters such as renal function and mortality. When meta-analyses were performed, these parameters appeared to go in the wrong direction and thus, set forth an enormous 5-year controversy regarding the use of this drug in clinical practice. The results of the ASCEND-HF trial are now available to answer important questions regarding this therapy, and confirm limited efficacy but clear safety.

The next 2 trials to come into the arena of acute decompensated heart failure were the Randomized Evaluations of Levosimendan (REVIVE) and Value of Endothelin Receptor Inhibition with Tezosentan in Acute Heart Failure Studies (VERITAS) programs, with the inodilator levosimendan and the vasodilator, neurohormonal, endothelin antagonist tezosentan.[5,6] The REVIVE program showed promise in that hemodynamics and symptom relief occurred early in the phase 2 studies. In fact, the phase 3 study, with a composite trichotomous in-hospital clinical endpoint of success, unchanged, or failure did indeed show clinical improvement. The mortality signal went in the opposite direction, thus precluding enthusiasm for regulatory approval in the United States, although individual countries in Europe have approved the drug.

The endothelin antagonist program starting with tezosentan was a development program that highlighted many of the challenges in developing AHF drugs. In phase 2 studies, there was evidence of hemodynamic improvement and a potential signal toward improved clinical outcomes of hospitalization plus death. However, when 4 systematic phase 2 studies were conducted, it was clear that the dose was high, and there appeared to be excessive sustained hypotension, resulting in renal insufficiency and even worsening in hospital heart failure. The investigations returned to phase 2 with a much smaller dose–response spectrum; cutting the dose almost tenfold still showed evidence of hemodynamic effect. This dose was then taken to a large phase 3 program of 2 nested trials. The primary endpoint was combined dyspnea relief and inhospital worsening heart failure or death. The program randomized approximately 900 patients, and was unsuccessful in demonstrating a benefit on the primary endpoint. Thus, the development program was terminated. Lessons learned from this trial included the complex issues of choosing a dose in phase 2, the uncoupling of hemodynamic changes with clinical outcomes, and the difficulty in modulating dyspnea compared with a usual care control group.

The next set of trials in the acute decompensated heart failure space were The Efficacy of Vasopressin Antagonism in Heart Failure

Outcome Study With Tolvaptan (EVEREST) and the Placebo-Controlled Randomized Study of the Selective A(1) Adenosine Receptor Antagonist Rolofylline for Patients Hospitalized With Acute Decompensated Heart Failure and Volume Overload to Assess Treatment Effect on Congestion and Renal Function (PROTECT) trials, with more novel approaches to managing fluid in these patients.[7–9] In the EVEREST trial, the vasopressin antagonist tolvaptan was studied in over 4000 patients to determine if there was an effect on morbidity and mortality. The basis of this drug development program was that tolvaptan was effective in providing enhanced aquaresis and free water fluid removal without electrolyte disturbances. It was postulated that this may be a better method for removing fluid in an acute decompensated heart failure patient compared with higher doses of furosemide, which had been associated with worse outcomes. In phase 2, there was a signal toward improved clinical outcomes and reduction in weight, which led to the larger EVEREST study. This consisted of 2 nested studies with short-term and long-term outcomes. The randomized, double-blind placebo-controlled trial demonstrated that there was no advantage on clinical outcomes, cardiovascular hospitalization, or death at a median follow-up of 9 months. In-hospital outcomes did achieve success on the primary outcome measure, which was a combination of weight plus patient global assessment. However, the components were divergent in which weight was indeed decreased, but the patient global assessment was neutral. A secondary endpoint of dyspnea showed an advantage for tolvaptan. The findings of this study revealed that indeed it was very difficult to beat usual care in the removal of fluid in these patients. While there was greater weight change in the tolvaptan group, this did not translate into improved hospitalization or death rates. Interestingly, the patient global assessment did not demonstrate improvement, although late dyspnea change was different between groups. Thus, lessons learned include at an early period in AHF, given greater clinical in-hospital improvement, that perhaps the choice of dyspnea as a primary endpoint would have been advantageous. Second, it is difficult to control for the diuretic dose in a placebo-controlled trial (ie, the tolvaptan-treated patients were initially getting the same doses of diuretics plus treatment, which could provide challenges with respect to preserving renal function and preventing other adverse events).

The PROTECT study targeted a more specific population of patients with acute decompensated heart failure who had some degree of renal insufficiency.[9] The hypothesis was that the adenosine A1 antagonist, roloffyline, could facilitate dieresis while also improving renal function, which would translate to improved clinical outcomes. Again, in the early phase studies the signals for improvement in renal function were strong. Thus, the 2000 patient PROTECT trial was conducted in a randomized, placebo-controlled study. Surprisingly, in this study, the renal function did not improve, and only approximately 10% to 12% of patients had a clinically important worsening renal function, which was the target of the therapeutic intervention. Again, perhaps misled by improper choice of endpoints, dyspnea was improved in this patient population, and perhaps should have been elevated to a primary endpoint status. There was no improvement in clinical outcomes at 60 days between the 2 groups, again perhaps reflecting the fact that the improvement in renal function was not seen. This also may reflect that the dose of the drug was not properly assessed in phase 2, and that the hypothesis that the drug improved renal function was based on a relatively small number of patients. It remains unclear, but re-emphasizes the point that phase 2 studies have to be more robust in the hypothesis testing, dose finding, and clinical signals.

Finally the most recent study, ASCEND-HF, enrolled 7148 patients in a randomized clinical trial of nesiritide versus placebo.[10] The coprimary endpoints were dyspnea at 6 and 24 hours, and rehospitalization for heart failure or death at 30 days. This landmark trial provides valuable information for future drug development in this field, as it demonstrates that indeed using global resources in an outcomes trial with sufficient power can be conducted in the acute decompensated heart failure setting. Proper endpoints can be ascertained globally, and enormous insight into drug mechanisms can be made by nesting in important substudies of biomarkers and other physiologic measurements.

In conclusion, phase 3 drug development in acute decompensated heart failure has experienced considerable evolution over the past decade by bringing the principles of clinical trials methodology into this field. Borrowed from the acute MI experience and other cardiovascular experiences, the field has matured to a point where proper conduct of phase 3 trials now has been set at the highest standard by incorporating the principles learned over decades of trials. This includes selection of patient populations, randomization process, double-blind methodology, and independent clinical endpoint assessments, with robust sample size calculations. However, given the lack of advancement in finding therapeutics that provide clinically meaningful benefit, further work needs to be done in the phase 1 and phase 2 arenas in this field to screen out molecules that will have a higher degree of success in phase 3 programs, given the complexity and expense of running these trials in this AHF population.

REFERENCES

1. Fonarow GC, Abraham WT, Albert NM, et al. Prospective evaluation of beta-blocker use at the time of hospital discharge as a heart failure performance measure: results from OPTIMIZE-HF. J Card Fail 2007;13:722–31.

2. Abraham WT, Adams KF, Fonarow GC, et al. In-hospital mortality in patients with acute decompensated heart failure requiring intravenous vasoactive medications: an analysis from the Acute Decompensated Heart Failure National Registry (ADHERE). J Am Coll Cardiol 2005;46:57–64.

3. Colucci WS, Elkayam U, Horton DP, et al. Intravenous nesiritide, a natriuretic peptide, in the treatment of decompensated congestive heart failure. Nesiritide Study Group. N Engl J Med 2000;343:246–53.

4. Cuffe MS, Califf RM, Adams KF Jr, et al. Short-term intravenous milrinone for acute exacerbation of chronic heart failure: a randomized controlled trial. JAMA 2002;287:1541–7.

5. Mebazaa A, Nieminen MS, Packer M, et al. Levosimendan vs dobutamine for patients with acute decompensated heart failure: the SURVIVE Randomized Trial. JAMA 2007;297:1883–91.

6. McMurray JJ, Teerlink JR, Cotter G, et al. Effects of tezosentan on symptoms and clinical outcomes in patients with acute heart failure: the VERITAS randomized controlled trials. JAMA 2007;298:2009–19.

7. Gheorghiade M, Gattis WA, O'Connor CM, et al. Effects of tolvaptan, a vasopressin antagonist, in patients hospitalized with worsening heart failure: a randomized controlled trial. JAMA 2004;291:1963–71.

8. Cotter G, Dittrich HC, Weatherley BD, et al. The PROTECT pilot study: a randomized, placebo-controlled, dose-finding study of the adenosine A1 receptor antagonist rolofylline in patients with acute heart failure and renal impairment. J Card Fail 2008;14:631–40.

9. Massie BM, O'Connor CM, Metra M, et al. Rolofylline, an adenosine A1-receptor antagonist, in acute heart failure. N Engl J Med 2010;363:1419–28.

10. O'Connor CM, Starling RC, Hernandez AF, et al. Effect of nesiritide in patients with acute decompensated heart failure. N Engl J Med 2011;365:32–43.

Clinical Trials in Mechanical Circulatory Support

Gregory Egnaczyk, MD, PhD[a,1], Carmelo A. Milano, MD[b],
Joseph G. Rogers, MD[a,c],*

KEYWORDS

- Mechanical circulatory support
- Left ventricular assist device • Bridge to transplant
- Destination therapy • Objective performance criteria

Discrepancy between the number of suitable organs available for cardiac transplantation and the burgeoning number of patients with advanced heart failure has driven the development, testing, and clinical application of left ventricular assist devices (LVADs) as an alternative treatment for this patient population. Over four decades of clinical investigation, many of the technical challenges associated with mechanical circulatory support (MCS) have been resolved by collaboration between talented engineers and clinician-scientists. The field of MCS has witnessed several critical paradigm shifts, including the transition from pneumatic to electrically driven pumps, the recognition that devices were not required to provide pulsatile blood flow, and the more recent implantation of LVADs in patients in whom there was no plan to remove the device (so-called "Destination Therapy" [DT]). The evolution of mechanically assisted circulation has resulted in improved device durability, reduction in pump size, fewer adverse events, and enhanced quality of life and survival. The pace of device refinement and transformation has been rightfully checked by careful and rigorous clinical evaluation in human subjects. Trial design, implementation, and interpretations have presented their own set of unique challenges.

This article discusses some of the challenges associated with LVAD trials as well as the evolution of LVAD trial design, using examples from prior and current studies.

DEFINING TREATMENT INTENT FOR LVADs

The "gold standard" therapy for patients with advanced heart failure remains heart transplantation. The number of heart transplants performed annually, however, has plateaued over the past decade despite a growing number of patients with advanced heart failure. The net result of this imbalance between potential transplant recipients and suitable donors is rationing of the therapy, prolonged waiting times, and clinical deterioration on the waiting list. The annual mortality of individuals listed for cardiac transplantation is approximately 17%.[1] Current heart allocation in the United States gives priority to the sickest individuals. Waiting for a patient's condition to worsen, a state often characterized by multiorgan dysfunction, has a negative impact on the perioperative survival of cardiac transplant recipients. Presensitization with anti-HLA antibodies, type O blood, and large body habitus further lengthens waiting times.[2] Given the uncertainty of donor availability

Funding support: None.
Financial disclosures: JGR, Thoratec, Consultant/Advisory Board, less than $10,000; CAM and GE, none.
a Division of Cardiology, Duke University Medical Center, Box 3034 DUMC, Durham, NC 27710, USA
b Division of Cardiothoracic Surgery, Duke University Medical Center, Box 3043 DUMC, Durham, NC 27710, USA
c Duke Clinical Research Institute, Box 3043 DUMC, Durham, NC 27710, USA
1 Address change as of January 1, 2011, The Christ Hospital, 2123 Auburn Avenue, Suite 139, Cincinnati, OH 45219.
* Corresponding author. Division of Cardiology, Duke University Medical Center, Box 3034 DUMC, Durham, NC 27710.
E-mail address: Joseph.rogers@duke.edu

Heart Failure Clin 7 (2011) 457–466
doi:10.1016/j.hfc.2011.06.005
1551-7136/11/$ – see front matter © 2011 Elsevier Inc. All rights reserved

and unpredictable, yet common, decompensation seen in these patients, there is a strong desire to stabilize patients while awaiting heart transplantation. This is the rationale behind use of LVADs as "Bridge to Transplant" (BTT).

LVADs were first used and tested in transplant candidates with rapidly deteriorating clinical and hemodynamic status. The advantages of studying mechanically assisted circulation in these high-risk patients were twofold: the potential benefit of circulatory support from LVADs matched the degree of risk, and the duration of support was predictably short. Re-establishment of end-organ perfusion and reduction of cardiac filling pressures reversed multiorgan failure and improved perioperative outcomes during subsequent cardiac transplantation.[3] Furthermore, patients were given time for nutritional and physical rehabilitation while supported on the device.

From a clinical trials perspective, the intent of BTT allowed for cardiac transplantation as a bailout if a device malfunction or complication arose. Restricted treatment intent translated, however, to fairly strict trial inclusion/exclusion criteria, a limited patient pool, and a small number of investigative sites. The net result was small trials that took many years to complete. Such were the limitations that faced clinical investigators in the 1980s and 1990s as they developed clinical experience in LVAD therapy.

The first successful use of LVAD as a BTT was reported in 1986 with a pneumatically driven device that tethered patients to a large console and limited patient mobility.[4] In 1991, implantation of the first intracorporeal left ventricular assist system (LVAS) launched a multicenter clinical evaluation of LVADs as a BTT using the HeartMate (HM) implantable pneumatic (IP) LVAS.[5] This small, nonrandomized trial compared outcomes of 34 patients who received an LVAD with 6 patients who met inclusion criteria but were managed with medical therapy in conjunction with an intra-aortic balloon pump. Survival to transplantation was 65% in the LVAD cohort with 80% of those patients discharged from the hospital. Fifty percent of the control group survived to transplantation but none survived beyond 77 days of reaching inclusion criteria for trial enrollment. The frequency of post-implant bleeding, infection, and right heart failure provided important insights regarding the adverse events that should be anticipated in the context of an LVAD trial. On the basis of this trial, the Food and Drug Administration (FDA) approved this device for BTT in 1994.

Advances in device and controller design technology at Thoratec (Pleasanton, California) resulted in the transition from the pneumatic device to a vented electric (VE) LVAD. The HM VE contained a textured polyurethane diaphragm and 25-mm porcine xenograft valves at both the inflow and outflow conduits. These surfaces reduced activation of the coagulation cascade and minimized the need for anticoagulation. A prospective, nonrandomized multicenter trial was conducted examining morbidity and mortality outcomes in 280 patients implanted with the HM VE as a BTT.[6] The historical control group for this trial consisted of 48 patients treated with optimal therapy. Survival to transplantation (67%) or recovery with device explantation (4%) in the LVAD patients exceeded those in the control group (33%). Mechanically supported patients had a 1-year post-transplant survival of 84%. On the basis of this study, a revised version of the HM VE (HM XVE) received FDA approval as a BTT in 1998.

The Novacor N100 (WorldHeart, Oakland, California) was another implantable electric pulsatile pump tested as a BTT. A single-center, prospective, nonrandomized study was performed comparing the Novacor LVAD to the HM VE as BTT.[7] Baseline characteristics and survival to transplant were similar between groups. More neurologic complications occurred with Novacor whereas infection and device malfunction were more frequent in the HM cohort. The Novacor LVAD also completed a BTT trial. Although never published, the results provided sufficient evidence to support FDA approval of this device for patients awaiting transplant. This device is no longer manufactured.

Refinement of patient selection criteria, surgical technique, and postoperative care coupled with technologic advances provided the rationale for studying LVADs for their original intent as permanent replacement of a diseased heart. The use of LVADs in patients deemed unsuitable for transplant is commonly referred to as DT. To test the efficacy of LVADs for DT in patients with advanced heart failure, the first multicenter randomized controlled trial (RCT) of LVADs was performed. The Randomized Evaluation of Mechanical Assistance for the Treatment of Congestive Heart Failure (REMATCH) trial randomized 129 patients with NHYA class IV heart failure who were not candidates for cardiac transplantation and had additional poor prognostic characteristics (left ventricular ejection fraction <25%, peak oxygen consumption <12 mL/kg/min, or inotrope dependence) to receive an HM VE LVAD or remain on optimal medical therapy.[8] Kaplan-Meier survival analysis demonstrated a significant 48% reduction in risk of death from any cause in the LVAD group (Fig. 1). The study also demonstrated an improvement in quality of life with the device group.

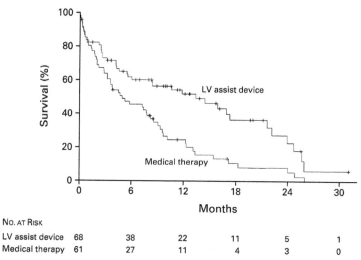

Fig. 1. Survival rates from the REMATCH trial. Kaplan-Meier survival curves in the group that received the HM VE LVAD and the group that received optimal medical therapy in the REMATCH trial.[7] Crosses depict censored patients. (*Reprinted from* Rose EA, Gelijns AC, Moskowitz AJ, et al. Long-term use of a left ventricular assist device for end-stage heart failure. N Engl J Med 2001;345:1435–45; with permission.)

Another clinically recognized indication for LVAD implantation is bridge to decision. This indication for mechanically supported circulation has not been examined in the context of a clinical trial. Restoration of a normal cardiac output and normalization of intracardiac filling pressures often results in resolution of contraindications to cardiac transplantation, including end-organ dysfunction and pulmonary hypertension, and allows the transplant center to acquire additional data on patient compliance and psychosocial stability.[9] It also allows additional time for patients to benefit from nutritional and physical rehabilitation. In such circumstances, individuals with contraindications to transplantation at the outset may ultimately become suitable transplant candidates.

Entry criteria for mechanical circulatory support trials in the United States continue to require declaration of intent for treatment (BTT vs DT) at the time of enrollment.[10] The practical consequences of this paradigm include relatively slow patient accrual in trials and delayed availability of new devices for clinical application. As LVAD technology and device durability have improved, criteria for trial success have been established, and costs of clinical trials have increased, development of novel trial designs are needed. These trials should define entry criteria based on the degree of cardiac dysfunction and physiologic derangements associated with heart failure rather than a future care pathway that may or may not occur. The intent of the device is less important than whether a patient requires mechanical support, would survive the perioperative period, and would have meaningful expected survival thereafter.

DEFINING THE CONTROL GROUP IN LVAD TRIALS

A critical component of any rigorous scientific investigation is the control group. The highest level of experimental validity occurs when baseline characteristics and conditions are identical in the intervention and control groups and the only meaningful difference between the cohorts is the intervention of interest. In clinical investigations, this is best approximated in RCTs. For approval of novel drug therapies, an RCT is a required component of the regulatory process. For approval of novel medical devices, RCTs are less commonly used. Several practical constraints have made the implementation of RCTs in evaluation of LVAD efficacy difficult. First, RCTs require equipoise. Until recently, LVAD trials have focused on patients with advanced heart failure and cardiogenic shock. These patients have annualized mortality rates of 80% to 90%.[11,12] There is no longer equipoise to randomize patients with this severity of illness to a strategy based on optimal medical therapy since improvements in quality of life and survival with mechanical circulatory support have been established. Second, patients and their families must be willing to accept the vicissitudes of randomization. Third, RCTs require a large sample size to ensure standard levels of power and allowance for type I error. Patient populations with advanced heart failure meeting trial inclusion/exclusion criteria and the number of centers with expertise in ventricular assist device trials are limited. Thus, the time to enroll acceptable patients in two arms of an RCT is lengthy. Finally, the rapid evolution of this field has resulted from an iterative relationship between clinicians and engineers. Small RCTs typically do not have the inherent flexibility to make changes to protocol or device.

Prospective observational trials circumvent many of the limitations of RCTs (described previously). Chiefly, single-arm nonrandomized trials decrease the number of patients required for enrollment. Through the use of historical data (historical control group, objective performance criteria, and registry-derived control group) and elimination of a concurrent control group, the sample size can be reduced by 75%.[13] Prospective observational trials can be more flexible in execution and adaptable to protocol changes and device modifications. The selection of prospective, observational studies as an alternative trial design to RCTs introduces many biases that make interpretation of the results challenging and conclusions less definitive. Hence, the choice of trial design involves a difficult balance between fostering innovation while maintaining rigor in evaluation and safety in implementation. **Table 1** lists the trials of LVADs over the years and delineates the trial design and the control group used in each study.

In prospective observational trials, definition of a control group provides a context for comparison. The goal is to select a group with patient characteristics that are similar to the treatment group. This strategy may result in case selection bias that is one of the great limitations of this type of trial design.[12] Historical controls for nonrandomized trials can be defined by one of two processes. A historical group may be created from a retrospective analysis of similar patients who would have met the inclusion and exclusion criteria for the trial in question (eg, BTT trial for HM VE LVAS). Objective performance criteria (OPC) are another variation of historical control. OPC are predetermined event rates, also known as performance goals, that if met allow the medical and regulatory communities to accept the device as effective and safe. OPC are based on broad sets of data from historical databases that are generally recognized as acceptable values. When using OPC, a new device must be demonstrated as not worse than the specified rates for the given endpoint within a margin of error.[14] For example, since 1994, the FDA has established OPC for use in single-arm trials of novel prosthetic heart valves. One potential advantage of OPC relative to the use of historical data from a prior clinical trial is the ability to continuously update the criteria based on new data from new trials.

REMATCH dramatically altered LVAD trial design.[15] The notion of a randomized trial for patients with advanced heart failure and cardiogenic shock had not previously been considered feasible. To ensure strict adherence to study entry criteria and background medical therapies, a gatekeeper was used to monitor and approve patients at the time of enrollment. More than 900 patients were screened for REMATCH before enrollment of the 129 who comprised the final randomized cohort. Background therapy included inotropic agents in approximately 75% of patients. The REMATCH trial demonstrated 1-year and 2-year survival rates of 25% and 8%, respectively, in the medically treated control group. Subsequent studies confirmed the poor performance of medical therapy in patients with this degree of illness. The INTrEPID study reported an 11% 1-year survival in inotrope-dependent patients and the Continuous Outpatient Support with Inotropes (COSI) study[11] showed a 6% 1-year survival in outpatients treated with chronic inotropic support.

Table 1
Select clinical LVAD trials with design characteristics

Trial/Device	Years of Enrollment	Indication	Trial Design	Control Group
HM IP LVAD	1985–1991	BTT	Prospective observational	Historical
HM VE LVAD	1996–1998	BTT	Prospective observational	Historical
HM VE (REMATCH)	1998–2001	DT	RCT	Medical therapy
INTrEPID	2000–2003	DT	Prospective observational	Medical therapy
HM II	2005–2006	BTT	Prospective observational	OPC
HM II	2005–2007	DT	RCT	HM XVE
VentrAssist	2004–2006	BTT	Prospective observational	OPC
HeartWare HVAD (ADVANCE-BTT)	2008–2010	BTT	Prospective observational	IDC
REVIVE-IT	2011–2016	DT	RCT	Medical therapy

Abbreviations: IDC, INTERMACS-derived concurrent cohort; OPC, objective performance criteria; XVE, modified vented electric.

Given the survival advantage associated with LVAD therapy, medical therapy is no longer considered a reasonable comparator group in patients with inotrope-dependent advanced heart failure. In this patient population, the equipoise had shifted to devices. For trials subsequent to REMATCH, evaluation of efficacy and safety of novel LVADs have been based on direct comparison with control groups of patients treated with previously approved devices or indirectly through a priori OPC set forth by the regulatory agencies.

As an example, the pivotal BTT trial for the continuous-flow LVAD, HM II, was designed as a nonrandomized single-arm study in which outcomes were compared with objective performance criteria.[16] The OPC for the primary endpoint (survival to transplantation or 180 days of device support) was 75%, a number based on historic and concurrent experience with LVAD therapy in the BTT application. Of 133 patients enrolled, 100 (75%) successfully reached the principal outcome. A continued-access protocol enrolled 336 additional patients before FDA approval of this device in 2008. An analysis of the first 281 patients who met study endpoints or completed follow-up through 18 months demonstrated that 222 (79%) successfully reached the primary combined endpoint of transplantation or device explantation for myocardial recovery or remained alive with ongoing LVAD support at 18-month follow-up.[17] The primary causes of death were sepsis (4% of patients), stroke (4%), and right heart failure (3%) or were device related (3%). Bleeding requiring transfusion (53% of patients) or surgery (26%) was the most common adverse event. Other important adverse events and their frequency in the total patient population were stroke (8.9%), device-related infection (16%), renal failure (11%), and right heart failure (19%). The adverse event rates were improved compared with BTT trials of pulsatile pumps, specifically the HM VE.[6] A total of 11 patients (4% of the cohort) underwent device replacement, none of which were due to a failure of the mechanical pumping mechanism. This also represented a significant improvement in reliability and durability over the pulsatile pumps. The probability of device failure at 24 months was 35% in the REMATCH trial with the HM VE[8] and 18% by 12 months in a retrospective analysis of patients implanted with the HM XVE.[18]

An example of a device versus device trial in a moribund population was the recently published HM II DT trial, an RCT comparing morbidity, mortality, and quality-of-life outcomes in patients randomized to a continuous-flow LVAD (HM II) or a pulsatile LVAD (HM XVE).[19] Two hundred patients

were enrolled, 134 patients in the continuous-flow cohort and 66 patients in the pulsatile-flow arm in concordance with the prespecified 2:1 ratio. The primary composite endpoint of survival free from disabling stroke and reoperation to repair or replace the LVAD at 2 years was successfully achieved by 46% of patients with continuous-flow devices as opposed to only 11% of patients with the pulsatile-flow pump, driven largely by reduction in the need to repair or replace the continuous-flow pump. Actuarial survival is shown in **Fig. 2**. In addition, the continuous-flow pump was associated with fewer adverse events, including sepsis, right heart failure requiring extended use of inotropes, respiratory failure, and renal failure. The rate of disabling stroke did not different differ statistically between the two groups (11% vs 12%).

The pivotal trial for the continuous-flow, centrifugal-flow VentrAssist LVAD (Ventracor, Chatswood, Australia) for Conformité Européene mark approval was implemented as a nonrandomized single-arm study.[20] The primary trial endpoint was survival to transplant or 154 days. The OPC for this primary endpoint was 65%. The trial enrolled 30 patients, of whom 25 met the primary endpoint for a success rate of 83%. The pivotal US trial for BTT approval completed enrollment but the results were not published and manufacturing of this device has ceased.

The HeartWare HVAD (HeartWare, Framingham, MA, USA) is currently undergoing clinical investigation in the US as a BTT. This continuous-flow, centrifugal-flow pump has gained Conformité Européene mark approval for use in Europe. The HeartWare HVAD is unique among LVADs in that the entire pump is contained within the pericardium, avoiding creation of a pump pocket in the abdominal wall. Data on the first 23 patients implanted with the device demonstrated that 91% successfully achieved the primary endpoint of survival to transplantation or continued device support at 180 days.[21] The US BTT trial with this device (ADVANCE-BTT) has completed enrollment. The trial was designed as a single-arm study with a contemporaneous control group derived from the Interagency Registry for Mechanically Assisted Circulatory Support (INTERMACS) (discussed later).

A recent strategy to define an appropriate control group is to derive the cohort from a multicenter, contemporaneous registry of patients supported with an approved LVAD. An appropriate registry would contain sufficient patients and data elements to allow advanced statistical methods, including propensity matching of trial and registry patients. Ideally this standardized data set would be

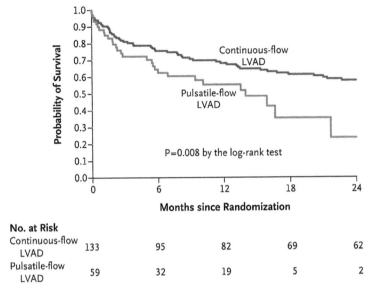

No. at Risk

Continuous-flow LVAD	133	95	82	69	62
Pulsatile-flow LVAD	59	32	19	5	2

Fig. 2. Survival rates of LVADs as DT. Kaplan-Meier survival curves in the group that received the pulsatile-flow LVAD (HM XVE) and the group that received the continuous-flow LVAD (HM II). (*Reprinted from* Slaughter MS, Rogers JG, Milano CA, et al. Advanced heart failure treated with continuous-flow left ventricular assist device. N Engl J Med 2009;361:2241–51; with permission.)

independent of the investigational device and would generate contemporaneous objective performance criteria. In 2006, through the joint efforts of the National Heart, Lung, and Blood Institute; the FDA; the Centers for Medicare & Medicaid Services; clinicians; and industry representatives, INTER-MACS was created. INTERMACS is a national registry intended to capture data on all noninvestigational mechanical circulatory support devices implanted with the intention of durable support. Participation in this national registry is required to obtain accreditation and reimbursement for implantation of LVADs. A critically important aspect of IN-TERMACS was the development of consensus definitions for adverse events. INTERMACS provides a rich data set reflective of the current practice of LVAD therapy in the United States as well as a control group of patients that can be extracted for comparison in trials of investigational devices.

In summary, there has been an evolution in trial design in the past decade of LVAD clinical investigation. The BTT trials have relied on nonrandomized single-arm trial to rapidly develop clinical experience with a novel pump design. The DT trials have used RCT design to rigorously support their use in a patient population ineligible for transplantation. As the field continues to progress and survival rates improve, it should be anticipated that patient selection criteria will be reassessed and less ill patients will be included in clinical trials. Furthermore, survival will play a less prominent role in endpoint selection and a natural transition

to functional and quality-of-life measures may become the primary focus of future trials with these devices.[22]

PATIENT SELECTION FOR TRIALS OF MECHANICALLY ASSISTED CIRCULATION

In the early years of their use, mechanical circulatory support was reserved for hospitalized patients failing medical therapy and treated with inotropic agents and intra-aortic balloon pumps. These patients were facing impending death and implantation of an LVAD constituted a heroic, final-hour intervention. Even as experience grew associated with the physiologic recovery and survival improvements seen with contemporary LVADs, the therapy was reserved for the sickest patients with refractory cardiogenic shock.

The HM VE BTT trial had stringent inclusion criteria. Aside from transplant candidacy, suitable patients were required to be treated with inotropic therapy, intra-aortic balloon pump (if possible), pulmonary capillary or left atrial pressure greater than 20 mm Hg with either systolic blood pressure less than 80 mm Hg or a cardiac index less than 2.0 l/min/m^2.[6] The REMATCH trial was designed to enroll an ambulatory patient population ineligible for transplant but actually enrolled the sickest cohort ever studied in a RCT of patients with heart failure (**Fig. 3**). The patients were older than prior LVAD trials (average age 68) and had severely depressed left ventricular ejection fractions (mean

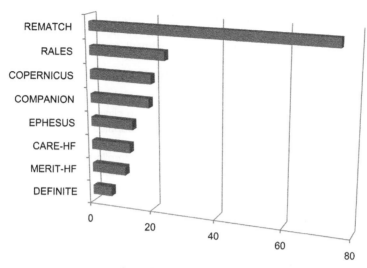

Fig. 3. Seven heart failure trials contemporary with execution of the REMATCH trial were examined. The annual mortality rate of the control group in each trial was plotted. REMATCH,[8] RALES,[30] COPERNICUS,[31] COMPANION,[32] EPHESUS,[33] CARE-HF,[34] MERIT-HF,[35] DEFINITE.[36] (Refs.[8,30–36])

17%) and a low cardiac index (mean 1.9 l/min/m²). Those well enough to undergo cardiopulmonary exercise testing had a peak oxygen consumption of only 9.18 ± 1.98 mL/kg/min. Approximately 70% of enrolled participants were unable to be weaned from inotropes and could not exercise.

Despite the dramatic survival benefit demonstrated in REMATCH, LVADs have only been tested in patients with medical refractory cardiogenic shock. The INTrEPID trial as well as the more contemporary HM II trials had similar patient baseline characteristics. Patients had severely depressed left ventricular ejection fractions (14%–17%), high pulmonary capillary wedge pressure (24–25 mm Hg), shock-range cardiac index (2.1 L/min/m²), low serum sodium (134–135 mmol/L), and high baseline creatinine (1.4–1.8) despite a large proportion of patients treated with either inotropic support of intra-aortic balloon counterpulsation.

Patient selection for mechanical support outside of clinical investigation mirrors that of the clinical trials. INTERMACS-designated profiles provide a higher level of granularity in describing patients with advanced heart failure than the New York Heart Association (NYHA) functional classes (**Table 2**).[23] Profiles 1 and 2 describe patients who are declining despite inotropes—a group with refractory cardiogenic shock with anticipated high mortality without rapid institution of additional support. An analysis of INTERMACS of LVAD recipients from June 2006 to September 2009 demonstrated that 70% of the 1092 primary

Table 2
INTERMACS profiles

Profile	Description	Time Frame for Intervention
1.	Critical cardiogenic shock	Needed within hours
2.	Progressive decline on inotropic support	Needed within a few days
3.	Stable but inotrope dependent	Elective over a period of weeks to few months
4.	Resting symptoms home on oral therapy	Elective over period of weeks to few months
5.	Exertion intolerant	Variable urgency, depends on maintenance of nutrition, organ function, and activity
6.	Exertion limited	Variable urgency, depends on maintenance of nutrition, organ function, and activity
7.	Advanced NYHA class III symptoms	Transplantation or circulatory support may not be currently indicated

LVAD implants were implanted in patients classified as INTERMACS profile 1 or 2.[24] The use of LVADs in these patients has important mortality implications. Patients in profiles 1 and 2 have significantly higher 1-year mortality rates than those in profile 3 (approximately 27% vs approximately 15%).

The stringent enrollment criteria of LVAD trials have identified a population of patients with extremely poor prognosis and end-organ dysfunction. Such patients are unstable and at high risk of short-term and intermediate-term morbidity and mortality. Some of the underlying processes leading to such morbidity and mortality may be irreversible regardless of whether mechanical circulatory support improves perfusion. It such a setting, the benefits of LVADs may be less robust.

Physiologic recovery and mortality reduction of these moribund patients with LVAD therapy should encourage clinical trialists to expand their use to patients with less severe illness. The trial and real-world experience with these devices demonstrates, however, that in a majority of cases, LVADs are reserved for unstable patients with refractory cardiogenic shock and multiorgan dysfunction. The task of judging the imminence of death is the critical skill in the equation of deciding appropriate candidates for LVAD therapy. Hemodynamic parameters (intracardiac pressures, cardiac index, and systolic blood pressure) are not statistically different across INTERMACS profiles 1 through 4. Therefore, these measurements neither help assign profiles nor provide risk stratification. The challenge of future trials is to move beyond this moribund patient population into a more ambulatory yet still functionally limited cohort of individuals with progressive heart failure. Several investigators have developed multivariable models to assist with selection of patients with sufficient severity of illness that provision of survival advantage could reasonably be anticipated.[25,26] In addition, modeling of clinical characteristics that predict post-LVAD right heart failure[27] and mortality[28,29] have been generated but not used prospectively in a clinical trial to select patients.

The Randomized Evaluation of VAD Intervention Before Inotropic Therapy (REVIVE-IT) pilot study will be introduced in 2011 to test the hypothesis that LVAD therapy will provide important and measurable improvements in survival, functional, and quality-of-life outcomes in patients with less advanced heart failure than previously studied. This National Institutes of Health–sponsored initiative will randomize 100 patients who are not treated with inotropes to LVAD therapy or optimal medical and electrical therapy. The inclusion and exclusion criteria are designed to define a population in whom there will be equipoise regarding the assigned treatment group.

SUMMARY

Trials of novel LVADs have posed unique challenges to clinical investigators. Dichotomizing the patient population into two groups (BTT and DT) for trial purposes decreased the number of potential trial enrollees from an already limited supply and has extended the time to study completion. Patients with modifiable contraindications to transplantation who did not meet the stringent criteria for DT trial inclusion were unable to benefit from the latest-generation device. LVAD development has benefited from the smaller patient numbers and flexibility provided in single-arm, nonrandomized trials. The generation of control groups for these single-arm trials continues to evolve and, with control groups derived from INTERMACS, more valid and rigorous comparisons can be made. The tremendous rates of mortality and morbidity in these trials speak to the patient population selected for these devices. As the devices demonstrate greater durability and adverse events are better prevented and managed, LVAD therapy is expected to expand to a less moribund patient population in whom survival and quality-of-life benefits may be more robust.

REFERENCES

1. Johnson MR, Meyer KH, Haft J, et al. Heart transplantation in the United States, 1999–2008. Am J Transplant 2010;10:1035–46.
2. Mancini D, Lietz K. Selection of cardiac transplantation candidates in 2010. Circulation 2010;122:173–83.
3. Aaronson KD, Eppinger MJ, Dyke DB, et al. Left ventricular assist device therapy improves utilization of donor hearts. J Am Coll Cardiol 2002;39:1247–54.
4. Hill JD, Farrar DJ, Hershon JJ, et al. Use of a prosthetic ventricle as a bridge to cardiac transplantion for postinfarction cardiogenic shock. N Engl J Med 1986;314:626–8.
5. Frazier OH, Rose EA, Macmanus Q, et al. Multicenter clinical evaluation of the HeartMate 1000 IP left ventricular assist device. Ann Thorac Surg 1992;53:1080–90.
6. Frazier OH, Rose EA, Oz MC, et al. Multicenter clinical evaluation of the HeartMate vented electric left ventricular assist system in patients awaiting heart transplantation. J Thorac Cardiovasc Surg 2001; 122:1186–95.
7. El-Banayosy A, Arusoglu L, Kizner L, et al. Novacor left ventricular assist system versus Heartmate vented electric left ventricular assist system as a long-term mechanical circulatory support device

in bridging patients: a prospective study. J Thorac Cardiovasc Surg 2000;119:581–7.

8. Rose EA, Gelijns AC, Moskowitz AJ, et al. Long-term mechanical left ventricular assistance for end-stage heart failure. N Engl J Med 2001;345:1435–43.

9. Nair PK, Kormos RL, Teuteberg JJ, et al. Pulsatile left ventricular assist device support as a bridge to decision in patients with end-stage heart failure complicated by pulmonary hypertension. J Heart Lung Transplant 2010;29:201–8.

10. Felker GM, Rogers JG. Same bridge, new destinations rethinking paradigms for mechanical cardiac support in heart failure. J Am Coll Cardiol 2006;47:930–2.

11. Hershberger RE, Nauman D, Walker TL, et al. Care processes and clinical outcomes of continuous outpatient support with inotropes (COSI) in patients with refractory endstage heart failure. J Card Fail 2003;9:180–7.

12. Rogers JG, Butler J, Lansman SL, et al. Chronic mechanical circulatory support for inotrope-dependent heart failure patients who are not transplant candidates: results of the INTrEPID Trial. J Am Coll Cardiol 2007;50:741–7.

13. Parides MK, Moskowitz AJ, Ascheim DD, et al. Progress versus precision: challenges in clinical trial design for left ventricular assist devices. Ann Thorac Surg 2006;82:1140–6.

14. Grunkemeier GL, Jin R, Starr A. Prosthetic heart valves: Objective Performance Criteria versus randomized clinical trial. Ann Thorac Surg 2006;82:776–80.

15. Rose EA, Moskowitz AJ, Packer M, et al. The REMATCH trial: rationale, design, and end points. Randomized Evaluation of Mechanical Assistance for the Treatment of Congestive Heart Failure. Ann Thorac Surg 1999;67:723–30.

16. Miller LW, Pagani FD, Russell SD, et al. Use of a continuous-flow device in patients awaiting heart transplantation. N Engl J Med 2007;357:885–96.

17. Pagani FD, Miller LW, Russell SD, et al. Extended mechanical circulatory support with a continuous-flow rotary left ventricular assist device. J Am Coll Cardiol 2009;54:312–21.

18. Dowling RD, Park SJ, Pagani FD, et al. HeartMate VE LVAS design enhancements and its impact on device reliability. Eur J Cardiothorac Surg 2004;25:958–63.

19. Slaughter MS, Rogers JG, Milano CA, et al. Advanced heart failure treated with continuous-flow left ventricular assist device. N Engl J Med 2009;361:2241–51.

20. Esmore D, Spratt P, Larbalestier R, et al. VentrAssist left ventricular assist device: clinical trial results and Clinical Development Plan update. Eur J Cardiothorac Surg 2007;32:735–44.

21. Wieselthaler GM, O Driscoll G, Jansz P, et al. Initial clinical experience with a novel left ventricular assist device with a magnetically levitated rotor in a multi-institutional trial. J Heart Lung Transplant 2010.

22. Stevenson LW, Couper G. On the fledgling field of mechanical circulatory support. J Am Coll Cardiol 2007;50:748–51.

23. Stevenson LW, Pagani FD, Young JB, et al. INTER-MACS profiles of advanced heart failure: the current picture. J Heart Lung Transplant 2009;28:535–41.

24. Kirklin JK, Naftel DC, Kormos RL, et al. Second IN-TERMACS annual report: more than 1,000 primary left ventricular assist device implants. J Heart Lung Transplant 2010;29:1–10.

25. Levy WC, Mozaffarian D, Linker DT, et al. The Seattle Heart Failure Model: prediction of survival in heart failure. Circulation 2006;113:1424–33.

26. Lund LH, Aaronson KD, Mancini DM. Validation of peak exercise oxygen consumption and the Heart Failure Survival Score for serial risk stratification in advanced heart failure. Am J Cardiol 2005;95:734–41.

27. Matthews JC, Koelling TM, Pagani FD, et al. The right ventricular failure risk score a pre-operative tool for assessing the risk of right ventricular failure in left ventricular assist device candidates. J Am Coll Cardiol 2008;51:2163–72.

28. Lietz K, Long JW, Kfoury AG, et al. Outcomes of left ventricular assist device implantation as destination therapy in the post-REMATCH era: implications for patient selection. Circulation 2007;116:497–505.

29. Ketchum ES, Moorman AJ, Fishbein DP, et al. Predictive value of the Seattle Heart Failure Model in patients undergoing left ventricular assist device placement. J Heart Lung Transplant 2010;29:1021–5.

30. Pitt B, Zannad F, Remme WJ, et al. The effect of spironolactone on morbidity and mortality in patients with severe heart failure. Randomized Aldactone Evaluation Study Investigators. N Engl J Med 1999;341:709–17.

31. Packer M, Fowler MB, Roecker EB, et al. Effect of carvedilol on the morbidity of patients with severe chronic heart failure: results of the carvedilol prospective randomized cumulative survival (COPERNICUS) study. Circulation 2002;106:2194–9.

32. Bristow MR, Saxon LA, Boehmer J, et al. Cardiac-resynchronization therapy with or without an implantable defibrillator in advanced chronic heart failure. N Engl J Med 2004;350:2140–50.

33. Pitt B, Remme W, Zannad F, et al. Eplerenone, a selective aldosterone blocker, in patients with left ventricular dysfunction after myocardial infarction. N Engl J Med 2003;348:1309–21.

34. Cleland JG, Daubert JC, Erdmann E, et al. The effect of cardiac resynchronization on morbidity and mortality in heart failure. N Engl J Med 2005;352: 1539–49.

35. Effect of metoprolol CR/XL in chronic heart failure: Metoprolol CR/XL Randomised Intervention Trial in Congestive Heart Failure (MERIT-HF). Lancet 1999; 353:2001–7.

36. Kadish A, Dyer A, Daubert JP, et al. Prophylactic defibrillator implantation in patients with nonischemic dilated cardiomyopathy. N Engl J Med 2004; 350:2151–8.

Behavioral Intervention, Nutrition, and Exercise Trials in Heart Failure

Ileana L. Piña, MD, MPH[a,*], Gerard Oghlakian, MD[b], Rebecca Boxer, MD[b]

KEYWORDS

- Lifestyle modifications • Heart disease • Heart failure
- Nutrition • Exercise • Behavioral intervention

With the ageing of the population and advances in acute treatment of ischemic events and surgical techniques for coronary artery and valvular heart disease, the prevalence of heart failure (HF) has been increasing. Lifestyle modifications are an integral part of preventing and treating most pathologic human conditions, and include behavioral modifications, diet, and exercise. Despite advances in medical and device therapy for HF, clinicians still hope that patients will adhere to nonpharmacologic interventions, some of which can actually improve symptoms and quality of life. This article reviews the role of these lifestyle modifications in preventing and treating HF.

NUTRITION, MICRONUTRIENTS, AND WEIGHT

The role of nutrition and diet in the prevention and management of HF is increasingly being recognized. The guidelines published to date target dietary and lifestyle interventions in treating cardiovascular risk factors, such as diabetes, hypertension, dyslipidemia, tobacco use, and obesity, without clear nutritional recommendations for patients with known HF.[1] Identifying a good nutritional regimen for these patients is often complicated by comorbidities and specific needs, such as involuntary weight loss, sodium restriction, water restriction, chronic kidney disease, and elevated glucose. Although the Framingham Heart Study showed increased incidence of HF with increasing body mass index (BMI) in both genders, independent of other known cardiac risk factors,[2] this concern relates to the less-symptomatic patients in whom prevention is a growing issue.

As the syndrome of HF progresses into the later stages and NYHA classes, weight loss and anorexia or early satiety become problematic. Patients with advanced HF may be hospitalized frequently, which is disruptive to nutritional plans and food preparation at home.[3] If patients are markedly deconditioned and physically impaired, food preparation becomes challenging, and eating packaged foods will add to any malnutrition, not to mention increase sodium intake. Patient history should include food intake and elicit symptoms of anorexia and any unintentional weight loss. The American Heart Association (AHA)/American College of Cardiology (ACC) HF Guidelines also implicate gut congestion and inflammatory mechanisms as contributory factors for altered metabolism and lowered food intake leading to cardiac cachexia.[4,5] At least one study reported cachexia as a predictor of poor outcomes.[6,7]

[a] Case Western Reserve University, Cleveland, OH, USA
[b] Harrington McLaughlin Heart and Vascular Institute, Case Medical Center, University Hospitals of Cleveland, Cleveland, OH, USA
* Corresponding author. Case Western Reserve University, Cleveland, Ohio 44106.
E-mail address: ilppina@aol.com

Heart Failure Clin 7 (2011) 467–479
doi:10.1016/j.hfc.2011.06.003
1551-7136/11/$ – see front matter. Published by Elsevier Inc

Ershow and Costello[8] recommend nutritional interventions tailored to the stages of HF described in the ACC/AHA Guidelines. **Table 1** depicts dietary goals and nutritional issues according to stage. Patients who are at the early stage A and B should be counseled about decreasing any risk factors for HF, such as obesity, hypertension, and hyperlipidemia. Patients with HF are considered likely to benefit from nutritional treatments described in the Institute of Medicine's (IOM's) report on "The Role of Nutrition in Maintaining Health in the Nation's Elderly," given that most patients are older and have multiple comorbidities.[9] Disease management programs that often include dietary counseling have been shown to reduce adverse events associated with HF, such as hospitalizations.[10–12] The ACC/AHA Guidelines for chronic HF state: "Use of nutritional supplements as treatment for HF is not indicated in patients with current or prior symptoms of HF and reduced LVEF. (*Level of Evidence: C*)."[4]

SODIUM AND FLUID

In the first National Health and Nutrition Examination Survey (NHANES) Epidemiologic Follow-Up Study, and after adjustment for known risk factors for HF, sodium intake was a strong independent risk factor for development of HF in obese men over a 19-year follow-up period.[13] Sodium restriction has become one of the most common recommendations given to patients with HF. Dietary indiscretion with high sodium intake can be the cause of as many as 30% of HF admissions.[14,15] Patients should be instructed on how to best restrict sodium, such as avoiding smoked meats or canned foods. The AHA/ACC Guidelines for Heart Failure specify: "Sodium restriction is recommended in symptomatic HF to prevent fluid retention. Although no specific guidelines exist, excessive intake of salt should be avoided. Patients should be educated concerning the salt content of common foods. Class of recommendation IIa, level of evidence C."[16]

Discussions concerning fluid intake have been more disparate. The AHA/ACC Guidelines state: "Fluid restriction of 1.5–2 L/day may be considered in patients with severe symptoms of HF especially with hyponatremia. Routine fluid restriction in all patients with mild to moderate symptoms does not appear to confer clinical benefit."[16]

VITAMINS AND MICRONUTRIENTS

Macronutrients include carbohydrates and fats. Micronutrients are defined as essential cofactors for energy transfer, biochemistry, and the physiology of the heart. It is certainly plausible that the micronutrient demands of a pathologic process such as HF are different from those of the normal myocardium. Several authors have proposed the importance of micronutrients in heart failure for both oxidative stress and calcium homeostasis.[17,18]

Vitamins are chemically unrelated organic compounds that are essential in small amounts for normal cellular metabolism. Vitamins (except vitamin D) cannot be synthesized by humans. Vitamin A and B carotene supplementation have shown no benefit in primary or secondary prevention of coronary heart disease. In a meta-analysis of antioxidants, beta carotene (n = 138,113) supplementation did not show benefit, and in fact showed a small increase in cardiovascular death and all-cause mortality. Similarly, vitamin E (n = 81,788) supplementation did not provide mortality benefit, reduction of cardiovascular death, or decrease in cerebrovascular accident.[19] In the Heart Outcomes Prevention Evaluation (HOPE) trial, vitamin E supplementation also showed no benefit, and in fact increased the risk of and hospitalization for heart failure.[20,21] Vitamin C supplementation has also shown no benefit in primary or secondary prevention of coronary heart disease. The best evidence includes the B vitamin family, carnitine, coenzyme Q10, and creatine. The more salient and best-studied micronutrients and vitamins are discussed.

Vitamin B

Thiamine (vitamin B_1) is water-soluble vitamin and is a coenzyme in carbohydrate metabolism. Absence of thiamine can cause wet beriberi with peripheral vasodilation and high output failure. Reports have shown that loop diuretic use can provoke thiamine loss.[22,23] Malnutrition and aging can also cause thiamine deficiency. In a study of 38 patients, 21% had biochemical evidence of low thiamine and 25% were at risk for insufficient thiamine according to dietary recall.[24] Deficiency was more common in patients with poor left ventricular function. In a study of hospitalized patients with HF, 33% had chemical thiamine deficiency compared with 12% of a control group. Patients with more advanced HF had the lowest thiamine levels. When lost in the urine, particularly with furosemide, nutritional ordinary amounts of thiamine may not be sufficient.[25]

Thiamine repletion studies have conflicted. Shimon and colleagues[26] supplemented patients who were on furosemide and compared them with a placebo group. The patients on thiamine showed measurable changes in ejection fraction of 22% and had increased diuresis. In contrast, another

Table 1
Nutritional issues and examples of dietary guidance for various stages of heart failure

Risk Group	ACC/AHA Stages of HF[30]	Dietary Goals (General)	Examples of Available Guidance	HF-Related Nutritional Issues
Low risk (Healthy general population)	N/A	*Primary prevention:* Keep risk factors in optimal range; achieve and maintain healthy weight and cardiovascular fitness	AHA Dietary Guidelines[1] Dietary Guidelines for Americans[76] Dietary Reference Intakes[75] WHO recommendations[72–74]	N/A
At risk of HF	*Stage A* At high risk for HF but without structural heart disease or symptoms of HF	*Primary prevention:* Achieve goals for management of risk factors or co-morbid conditions (hypertension, obesity, dyslipidemia, diabetes, alcohol use)	AHA Dietary Guidelines[1] DASH Diet (NHLBI)[77] TLC Diet (NHLBI)[78]	CVD risk factors Diabetes Kidney disease
	Stage B Structural heart disease but without signs or symptoms of HF	*Secondary prevention:* Achieve goals for management of risk factors after MI or other predisposing condition	AHA Dietary Guidelines[1] DASH Diet (NHLBI)[77] TLC Diet (NHLBI)[78]	Co-morbidities Overweight and obesity Sodium intake Alcohol intake
Diagnosis of HF	*Stage C* Structural heart disease with prior or current symptoms of HF	Maintain functional status and quality of life: Meet nutritional requirements; control symptoms; lessen need for medications; reduce progression of disease	As above, adding as needed: medical nutrition therapy for co-morbid conditions; dietary supplements Nutrition Screening Initiative Guidelines[79] ACC/AHA Guidelines[4] ESC Guidelines[16]	Drug-nutrient interactions Weight monitoring Fluid retention Reduced exercise tolerance Sodium intake Alcohol intake
	Stage D Refractory HF requiring specialized interventions	Maintain functional status and quality of life: Meet nutritional requirements; control symptoms; minimize acute exacerbations and hospitalizations	As above, adding as needed: medical nutrition therapy for co-morbid conditions; dietary supplements; and enteral or parenteral nutritional support Nutrition Screening Initiative Guidelines[79] ACC/AHA Guidelines[4] ESC Guidelines[16]	Cachexia Transplantation medications Implantable devices Surgical nutrition issues Gastrointestinal function Fluid restriction

Abbreviations: AHA/ACC, American Heart Association/American College of Cardiology; CVD, cardiovascular disease; ESC, European Society of Cardiology; HF, heart failure; MI, myocardial infarction; N/A, not applicable; WHO, World Health Organization.
From Ershow AG, Costello RB. Dietary guidance in heart failure: a perspective on needs for prevention and management. Heart Fail Rev 2006;11:7–12; with permission.

study of 50 patients with decompensated HF failed to show improvements in dyspnea score or duration of hospitalization.[27] Further clinical trials are needed to examine the administration of thiamine in various groups of patients with HF, especially those with high diuretic requirements.

Riboflavin (vitamin B_2) and pyridoxine (vitamin B_6) are also water-soluble and excreted by the kidney and are dependent on intake. Keith and colleagues[28] studied 100 consecutive patients admitted for HF and compared them with a group without HF. Overall, 27% had biochemical evidence of vitamin B_2 deficiency, whereas 38% had evidence of B_6 deficiency. These rates were higher than in volunteers without HF. Biochemical evidence of at least one B vitamin was present in 68% of patients compared with 42% of volunteers. Vitamin supplementations resulted in a 50% lowering of deficiency rates for both vitamins B_2 and B_6, but these rates did not significantly differ from those in volunteers who did not take supplementation.

Homocysteine

Acknowledging the relationship between oxidative stress, left ventricular remodeling, and homocysteine-induced injury, Vasan and colleagues[29] examined the Framingham cohort over the decades of 1979 to 1982 and 1986 to 1990, who were initially free of any HF or myocardial infarction at baseline, and measured the incidence of HF over an 8-year period. Levels of homocysteine above the median value for gender were associated with a hazard ratio for HF of 1.93 in women and 1.84 in men, and the investigators concluded that increased homocysteine level was an independent predictor of the development of HF in individuals without previous myocardial infarction. To better identify the risk for HF and the relationship of homocysteine to other HF markers, such as echocardiographic parameters and B-type natriuretic protein (BNP), Herrmann and colleagues[30] studied 95 patients with New York Heart Association (NYHA) class II and III HF and found a correlation between homocysteine levels and severity of symptoms and levels of proBNP (**Fig. 1**). Both of these studies use a homocysteine level of 12 μmol/L as a cutoff for a higher risk, and therefore both of these studies are consistent.

Generally, deficiency of vitamins B_{12} or B_6, or folate is the most common cause of elevated levels of homocysteine. Supplements of these vitamins can be used to treat homocysteinemia, and are inexpensive. However, no studies relate vitamin B_{12} or B_6 (except as noted earlier) with HF.[30] Certainly further studies of supplementation in patients with elevated homocysteine levels and

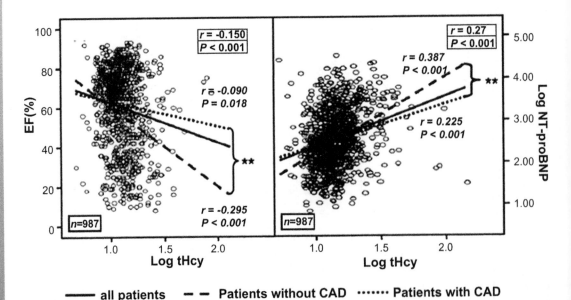

Fig. 1. Pearson's correlation analysis of logarithmically transformed (log) total homocysteine (tHcy) and left ventricular ejection fraction (EF) and log N-terminal pro-B-type natriuretic-peptide (NT-proBNP). The larger r and P values in the upper right corner of each plot represent the overall analysis including all patients. The smaller r and P values close to the lines are the results of the separate analyses for patients with and without coronary artery disease. **Significant difference between patients with and without coronary artery disease; P<.01 (multivariate regression analysis). (*From* Herrmann M, Muller S, Kindermann I, et al. Plasma B vitamins and their relation to the severity of chronic heart failure. Am J Clin Nutr 2007;85:117–23; with permission.)

changes in HF status could have significant implications on public health if positive.

Vitamin D

Evidence remains equivocal regarding the benefits of vitamin D supplementation in HF. The association of vitamin D deficiency and HF is shown in a variety of studies that demonstrate the translational aspect of this area of research. Vitamin D receptor knock-out mice showed increased expression of renin and angiotensin, resulting in hypertension and myocardial hypertrophy.[31] Laboratory studies have also shown that the vitamin D receptor is present on cardiac myocytes and that vitamin D opposes cell proliferation and can have an antihypertrophic effect.[32,33] The active form of vitamin D (1,25-dihydroxyvitamin D(3) [1,25(OH)D]) caused decreased renin expression.

Clinically, in patients with NYHA class II and III HF, lower vitamin D concentrations have been associated with lower functional capacity measured by both a shorter 6-minute walk and lower peak oxygen consumption per minute (VO_2) on cardiopulmonary stress testing, and with frailty.[34,35] The relationship between vitamin D and the health of skeletal muscle is of particular interest because of the chronic skeletal muscle loss and debilitation associated with HF. The traditional role of vitamin D is maintenance of calcium homeostasis and has long been known to be important to the health of the musculoskeletal system. Vitamin D can increase uptake of calcium, which may increase contractile force and increase muscle cell proliferation and differentiation. Vitamin D deficiency can result in a reversible myopathy characterized by muscle weakness, decreased muscle mass, and falls.[36–38]

Most evidence indicating a relationship between vitamin D deficiency in particular and heart failure is from observational studies. A recent analysis of the NHANES database indicates that patients with low serum 1,25(OH)D concentrations have an increased risk of all-cause mortality and death from HF.[39] Vitamin D concentrations were also found to be associated with mortality for patients with end-stage HF awaiting transplantation.[40] Patients referred for angiography had an increased risk of death from HF, or from sudden cardiac death in those with very low vitamin D concentrations.[41]

Few clinical trials of vitamin D therapy have been performed in patients with HF. A recent trial of patients with HF given 200,000 IU of vitamin D in divided doses over 10 weeks showed no effect on the 6-minute walk test or on quality of life.[42]

The 1,25(OH)D concentrations achieved in this trial may have been too low to have a physiologic affect, increasing baseline levels only by 9.2 ng/mL. Another trial showed that patients with HF who were given 2000 IU of vitamin D with calcium experienced an improvement in the inflammatory milieu compared with those given calcium alone for 9 months, but no difference in the rate of events was seen between the groups.[43] Further research is needed regarding the adequate amounts of vitamin D supplementation in patients with HF and to examine the hard end points of mortality and morbidity. The public health impact of an easily obtainable and inexpensive therapy could be significant.

BEHAVIOR
Collaborative Care

Patient self-management has taken center stage for programs dedicated to HF. More than 40% of hospitalizations caused by decompensated HF are related to patient behavior regarding nonadherence to diet or medication regimens.[15] Therefore, disease management programs concentrate much of their efforts on patient education.[44] However, patient education alone cannot alter patient behavior. The daily responsibilities of caring for a chronic illness rest with the patients themselves and their caregivers. Clinicians often forget that patients are the experts of their own lives and their priorities.

For patients to adhere to any therapy, diet, or drug, they must believe in the therapy or that what the clinician is saying is true. Entering the decision to be adherent also depends on the patients' subjective perception of risks versus benefits. A discussion of theories of behavior are outside of the scope of this article, but are addressed elsewhere.[45–47] None of these behaviors has been conclusively linked to HF management. Nonetheless, the concept of chronic care, such as in HF, must change from a model involving a provider prescribing to the patient and the patient passively receiving the information to one of collaborative care.[48] Collaborative care implies a relationship between provider and patient that supports self-management. In collaborative care, providers and patients make decisions about the care together. Self-management education must occur together with collaborative care through arming patients with the skills needed to better manage their disease within their lifestyle.

A pertinent example in HF care can be the flexible diuretic regimen, which allows patients to adjust their diuretic dose within a set of instructions by weight. This empowerment removes the patient's "conscience" concerns when they "misbehave" on their sodium intake by giving them the tools to prevent or treat an increase in weight. **Table 2** depicts descriptors of traditional care and collaborative care for HF. Collaborative care includes definition of problems together, targeting and goal setting, setting of realistic objectives, a continuum of self-management training and support, and active sustained follow-up with patient monitoring. Although this approach has been used mainly in asthma and diabetes, these concepts fit easily into HF chronic care.[48,49] Although disease management programs, all of which incorporate some form of patient education, have been successful in reducing hospitalizations, the impact on survival has been less well studied. More recently, the Heart Failure Adherence and Retention Trial (HART) compared patient self-management skills training in combination with HF education and HF education alone on the composite end points of death/HF hospitalizations and death/all-cause hospitalizations in patients with mild to moderate HF, whether with systolic dysfunction or preserved systolic function.[50]

Overall, 902 patients were randomized to receive patient education alone versus patient education and self-management counseling. No benefit was noted between groups in the combined end point of all-cause death or HF hospitalization over 2.56 years of follow-up. The event rate was high at 18.4% annually (**Fig. 2**). The only significant interaction between treatment and a prespecified risk factor analysis was patient income. Among patients with incomes less than $30,000, those randomized to receive self-management counseling were slower to have an event.[51] This finding, although in a post-hoc analysis, indicates a need to stratify patient education methodologies according to socioeconomic status or income in future trials.

Adherence

Adherence has been defined by Haynes and colleagues[52] as "the extent to which a person's behavior in terms of taking medications, following diets, or executing lifestyle changes coincides with medical or health advice." The World Health

Table 2
Comparison of traditional and collaborative care

Issue	Traditional Care	Collaborative Care
What is the relationship between patient and health professionals?	Professionals are the experts who tell patients what to do Patients are passive	Shared expertise with active patients Professionals are experts about the disease and patients are experts about their lives
Who is the principal caregiver and problem solver? Who is responsible for outcomes?	The professional	The patient and professional are the principal caregivers; they share responsibility for solving problems and for outcomes
What is the goal?	Compliance with instructions Noncompliance is a personal deficit of the patient	The patient sets goals and the professional helps the patient make informed choices Lack of goal achievement is a problem to be solved by modifying strategies
How is behavior changed?	External motivation	Internal motivation Patients gain understanding and confidence to accomplish new behaviors
How are problems identified?	By the professional (eg, changing unhealthy behaviors)	By the patient (eg, pain or inability to function; and by the professional)
How are problems solved?	Professionals solve problems for patients	Professionals teach problem-solving skills and help patients in solving problems

From Bodenheimer T, Lorig K, Holman H, et al. Patient self-management of chronic disease in primary care. JAMA 2002;288:2469–75; with permission.

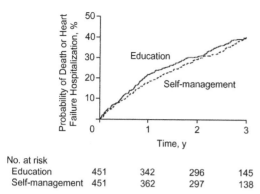

Fig. 2. Time to death or hospitalization from heart failure according to treatment group. (*From* Powell LH, Calvin JE Jr, Richardson D, et al. Self-management counseling in patients with heart failure: the heart failure adherence and retention randomized behavioral trial. JAMA 2010;304:1331–8; with permission.)

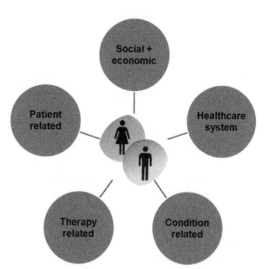

Fig. 3. Adherence: a multidimensional interplay. (*Adapted from* WHO. Adherence to long-term therapies: evidence for action. 2003. Available at: http://www.who.int/chp/knowledge/publications/adherence_full_report.pdf; with permission.)

Organization (WHO) modified this definition by adding "the extent to which a person's behaviour – taking medication, following a diet, and/or executing lifestyle changes, corresponds with agreed recommendations from a health care provider."[53] The alteration of this definition highlights the issue of joint decision making rather than a patient's passive acceptance of a provider's recommendations. A strong differentiation should be made between adherence and compliance. Adherence essentially requires the patient to agree to the recommendations. The WHO's report on adherence addresses chronic diseases. Although HF was not included, the definition of chronic diseases fits HF well. "Diseases which have one or more of the following characteristics: they are permanent, leave residual disability, are caused by nonreversible pathological alteration, require special training of the patient for rehabilitation, or may be expected to require a long period of supervision, observation or care."[53] Adherence is a multidimensional phenomenon affected by many factors in addition to those that are patient-related. Clinicians often blame patients for their failure to adhere to therapy, and thereby misunderstand other factors that also enter into the complexity of observed behavior. **Fig. 3** illustrates five of those factors or dimensions.

The importance and complexity of adherence is highlighted in the WHO report, with **Box 1** listing some important messages that are easily applied to the chronic care of patients with HF.

Because facilitating knowledge is a key aspect to seeking adherence, helpful points are noted in **Box 2**.

Perhaps facilitating self-efficacy (ie, the ability to see oneself in a place and time or in an activity and behavior) is the most difficult of all. **Box 3** includes tools to improve empowerment and build self-efficacy in patients with HF.

The importance of adherence cannot be better illustrated than in the HF-ACTION trial (Heart Failure: A Controlled Trial Investigating Outcomes Exercise Training) in which 2331 patients with NYHA class II through IV systolic HF were randomized to a program of exercise training or usual care. Both groups received patient education and excellent medical therapy. Patients randomized to exercise had multiple barriers facilitated for them – training sessions were free, the sites provided the parking and transportation, the sites found satellite centers for exercise convenient to the patients' home, and either a treadmill or bike was delivered to the patients' home when the home phase began. Phone calls, diaries, pulse-measuring monitors, and the ability to return to the exercise center for more sessions were among the approaches to encouraging exercise. Despite a high level of safety, adherence worsened as the trial ensued, and at best was approximately 40%. The results of the trial were modest and nonsignificant.[54] The challenges the trial investigators faced in achieving better adherence may have ultimately affected the results of the trial. Further analyses are ongoing to examine adherence to trial end points.

EXERCISE

The syndrome of HF becomes more evident when patients cannot perform activities initially at a higher work level, gradually worsening to inability to perform lower-level activities, and finally to

---

Box 1
Important points regarding adherence for patients with heart failure

- Poor adherence to the treatment of chronic diseases is a worldwide problem of striking magnitude.
- The impact of poor adherence increases as the burden of chronic disease increases worldwide.
- The consequences of poor adherence to long-term therapies are poor health outcomes and increased health care costs.
- Improving adherence also enhances patients' safety.
- Adherence is an important modifier of health system effectiveness.
- Increasing the effectiveness of adherence interventions may have a far greater impact on the health of the population than any improvement in specific medical treatments.[52]
- Health systems must evolve to meet new challenges.
- Patients must be supported, not blamed.
- Adherence is simultaneously influenced by several factors.
- Patient-tailored interventions are required.
- Adherence is a dynamic process that must be followed up.
- Health professionals must be trained in adherence.
- Family, community, and patients' organizations are key factors for success in improving adherence.
- A multidisciplinary approach toward adherence is needed

Box 2
Strategies to facilitate knowledge

- Identify and provide information where knowledge gaps exist.
- Discuss treatment goals.
- Demonstrate appropriate techniques for administering medication.
- Confirm understanding; have patient repeat information.
- Ask about concerns regarding medication uptake.
- Provide written information.
- Follow-up and monitor to reinforce information.

From Bucci KK, Possidente CJ, Talbot KA, et al. Strategies to improve medication adherence in patients with depression. Am J Health Syst Pharm 2003;60(24): 2601–5; with permission.

---

fact no relation exists between ejection fraction and exercise duration or between ejection fraction and oxygen uptake when measured with cardiopulmonary testing (CPX).[55] Therefore, the limitations to performing exercise are multifactorial and involve more than the central circulation,[56] which is why it is important to actually test exercise

---

Box 3
Tools to motivate and build confidence

Motivate

- Involve patient in problem-solving
- Provide information and alternatives
- Express empathy
- Avoid arguments
- Point out discrepancy between patient's behavior and important personal goals
- Involve family members
- Refer to support group

Build self-efficacy

- Enhance confidence to overcome barriers and succeed
- Recognize small positive steps
- Use supportive statements
- Help set reasonable and reachable goals
- Express belief that goals may be achieved

Data from World Health Organization. Adherence to long-term therapies: evidence for action. Available at: http://www.who.int/chp/knowledge/publications/adherence_full_report.pdf; with permission.

---

experiencing symptoms at rest. This inability to perform even daily living activities is what brings patients to the attention of clinicians. In addition, patients often decrease the activities that provoke symptoms or take a longer time to perform those activities. Similarly, nocturnal symptoms can be frightening and trigger a visit to a physician. HF can be defined as the inability of the heart to meet the oxygen and nutrient demands of the tissues, resulting in symptoms of fatigue or dyspnea on exertion that progress to dyspnea at rest. Therefore, exercise intolerance is tightly linked to the diagnosis of HF. A thorough history should uncover not only symptoms but also changes in activity pattern, duration, and frequency. One would expect that resting ventricular function would be predictive of functional capacity, but in function in patients with HF, because a resting ventricular function testing will not predict exercise response. Although CPX testing is the most direct and accurate measure of functional capacity and the oxygen uptake is related to prognosis, much can be learned from performing an exercise test without gas exchange. **Box 4** lists areas of abnormal circulatory response to exercise exhibited by patients with HF. Not all patients will be limited by the same factors. More extensive discussions of sources of exercise intolerance, including cardiac output, peripheral blood flow, muscle fibers, and oxidative metabolism have been reviewed elsewhere.[56–61]

Deconditioning and Bed Rest

As patients develop symptoms and are likely to be hospitalized, deconditioning can worsen with each admission. Moreover, family, friends, or even providers may have warned patients not to exercise so as not to "worsen" their failing heart. However, bed rest is detrimental to normals and much more so to patients with HF.[62,63] Patients with HF have inherent skeletal muscle abnormalities, and bed rest will worsen their muscle function. Other changes, such as an increase in maximal heart rate and a drop in vagal tone, will adversely affect HF even in medicated patients. Therefore, patients must attempt to maintain function as much as possible when at home and activity should be recommended as part of the nonpharmacologic treatment of HF.

Benefits of Exercise Training

The benefits of exercise training in patients with HF include an improvement in exercise tolerance as assessed not only by exercise duration but also more importantly by peak oxygen uptake (peak

V_{O_2}) as measured by CPX. Exercise training programs in studies have varied among supervised or home training; treadmill or bicycle; duration of 8 weeks to 3 months; and various levels of intensity from low to moderate. Changes in peak V_{O_2} have ranged from 12% to 31%. Most of the improvement occurs by week 3 but can still be noted at 6 months if compliance with the training program continues. Improvement is seen not only in maximal exercise performance but also in indices of submaximal exercise.[64–68] One can hypothesize that exercise training can improve flow-dependent relaxation of peripheral arteries, and that this beneficial effect can translate into an increased blood flow to skeletal muscles. In addition, an improvement in endothelium-dependent vasodilation of epicardial vessels and in resistance vessels in patients with known coronary artery disease has been shown after only 4 weeks of training, with the exercise group increasing coronary artery flow reserve by 29% compared with a nonexercise control group.[69]

Exercise training has also been shown to improve health status, including quality of life. In the HF-ACTION trial, the group undergoing exercise improved their score on the Kansas City Cardiomyopathy Questionnaire by the third month after randomization, and maintained this level throughout the first year.[70]

Safety

The HF-ACTION trial reported on the safety of exercise training, showing no difference in adverse events between the groups. The trial did not demand monitoring and left the election of electrocardiogram monitoring at the discretion of the training sites. The safety aspects of training were noticeable in the supervised early sessions and during continued exercise at home.[54]

Mortality and Hospitalizations

Most of the early trials included small numbers of patients, and were not powered to examine the hard end points of outcomes, including mortality and hospitalizations. The HF-ACTION trial directly studied these hard end points in patients randomized to either exercise or a control group consisting of patient education and excellent medical therapy. The study showed a modest nonsignificant reduction in the primary end point of all-cause mortality or all-cause hospitalization, and a modest but significant reduction when adjusted for key prognostic factors. (HR, 0.93; 95% CI, 0.84, 1.02; $P = .13$. Adjusted HR, 0.89; 95% CI, 0.81, 0.99; $P = .03$). The secondary end point of cardiovascular mortality or cardiovascular

---

Box 4
Sources of potential exercise limitations in heart failure

- Cardiac output
- Left ventricular end-diastolic pressure
- Left ventricular end-diastolic diameter and end-systolic diameter
- Peripheral reserve
- Chronotropic incompetence (may be related to a lower workload)
- Neurohormonal levels
- Respiratory muscle function
- Malnutrition
- Skeletal muscle changes

hospitalization did not show a significant difference between groups (HR, 0.92; 95% CI, 0.83, 1.03; $P = .14$. Adjusted HR, 0.91; 95% CI, 0.82, 1.01; $P = .09$). However, the secondary end point of cardiovascular mortality or HF hospitalization was nearly significant when unadjusted and significant when adjusted (HR, 0.87; 95% CI, 0.75, 1.00; $P = .06$. Adjusted HR, 0.85; 95% CI, 0.74, 0.99; $P = .03$).[54] Because of this interesting finding, and given the suboptimal adherence of the exercise group, further analyses are ongoing to determine the relationship of adherence to the end points. Therefore, exercise can be recommended as an adjunct to optimal medical therapy because of its safety, relation to improved health status, and modest reductions in end points.

Exercise Prescription

Because no agreement exists on a universal exercise prescription for patients with HF, an individualized approach is recommended. Exercise training guidelines for patients with cardiovascular disease should be followed as provided in the AHA standards.[71] Baseline exercise testing can be performed with or without gas exchange using protocols that optimize the estimation of functional capacity, such as through approaching a true maximum heart rate. No fixed protocol for testing is available, although the Modified Naughton has been more commonly used in studies. As in any exercise prescription, the components are intensity, duration, frequency, and progression. Progression should be included to allow the rehabilitation team to further the patient along a conditioning path.

Intensity
Intensity is defined as the workload to be imposed on the patient. Heart rate–derived exercise prescriptions may be inaccurate in patients with more advanced disease. In these patients, chronotropic reserve may be limited. In the current era of

ß-blockers, heart rate alone as a measure of intensity may not be practical. The most frequently used intensity range has been 70% to 80% of peak capacity determined in a symptom-limited (but of sufficient effort) exercise test. Very debilitated patients, or those who are not accustomed to aerobic activity, may need to initiate the program at a lower intensity (eg, 60% or 65% of peak capacity) and perform interval training with periods of rest. Progression must be built into the prescription to allow the rehabilitation staff to adjust the exercise intensity as the patient becomes better conditioned. The Borg scale can also be useful in prescribing exercise intensity especially in patients on ß-blockers. Intensities of 12 to 13 rate of perceived exertion (mild to moderate work) are usually well tolerated by stable patients. In the HF-ACTION trial, the heart rate reserve was used at 70% target. Patients early in the exercise phase started at 60% heart rate reserve and increased from there depending on their state of conditioning. This intensity was safe even in patients with more advanced disease. The same intensity was recommended in the home phase of the program.

Duration
Duration of exercise should include an adequate warm-up period. The warm-up may need to be longer in the most debilitated patients and can involve stretching, walking, or pedaling without resistance at lower revolutions per minute. Usually 10 to 15 minutes is recommended. The exercise duration most frequently used is 20 to 30 minutes at the desired intensity. A period of cool down is also advised. As noted in **Table 3**, the recommended duration in HF-ACTION was 30 to 35 minutes. As with intensity, a shorter duration can be used at the beginning of the program and gradually progressed.

Frequency
The most commonly recommended frequency of exercise is three to five times per week. Patients

Training Phase	Location	Week[a]	Sessions/ Week	Aerobic Minutes	Intensity (% Heart Rate Reserve)	Training Mode
Initial supervised	Clinic	1–2	3	15–30	60%	Walk/cycle
Supervised	Clinic	3–6	3	30–35	70%	Walk/cycle
Supervised and home	Clinic and home	7–12	3 and 2	30–35	70%	Walk/cycle
Maintenance	Home	13–end	5	40	60%–70%	Walk/cycle

Table 3
HF-ACTION: exercise training program

[a] Week intervals shown are goals and may vary for individual participants.

who develop exhaustion after training may need a day of rest between sessions. Supplemental walking should be encouraged. Patients with HF may experience fatigue after exercise training, but this usually dissipates as training ensues. Supervision is best, especially during initial training sessions. Home training can follow this early supervised period, which may vary among patients, depending on the level of deconditioning and disease stability. In the HF-ACTION trial, the initial phase consisted of three times per week followed by home training at five sessions per week.

REFERENCES

1. Lichtenstein AH, Appel LJ, Brands M, et al. Diet and lifestyle recommendations revision 2006: a scientific statement from the American Heart Association Nutrition Committee. Circulation 2006;114:82–96.
2. Kenchaiah S, Evans JC, Levy D, et al. Obesity and the risk of heart failure. N Engl J Med 2002;347:305–13.
3. Pasini E, Opasich C, Pastoris O, et al. Inadequate nutritional intake for daily life activity of clinically stable patients with chronic heart failure. Am J Cardiol 2004;93:41A–3A.
4. Hunt SA, Abraham WT, Chin MH, et al. 2009 focused update incorporated into the ACC/AHA 2005 Guidelines for the Diagnosis and Management of Heart Failure in Adults: a report of the American College of Cardiology Foundation/American Heart Association Task Force on Practice Guidelines: developed in collaboration with the International Society for Heart and Lung Transplantation. Circulation 2009;119(14):e391–479.
5. Delafontaine P, Akao M. Angiotensin II as candidate of cardiac cachexia. Curr Opin Clin Nutr Metab Care 2006;9:220–4.
6. Celik T, Yaman H. Elevated adiponectin levels in patients with chronic heart failure: An independent predictor of mortality or a marker of cardiac cachexia? Int J Cardiol 2009;144(2):319–20.
7. Shirley S, Davis LL, Carlson BW. The relationship between body mass index/body composition and survival in patients with heart failure. J Am Acad Nurse Pract 2008;20:326–32.
8. Ershow AG, Costello RB. Dietary guidance in heart failure: a perspective on needs for prevention and management. Heart Fail Rev 2006;11:7–12.
9. Institute of Medicine (U.S.). Committee on Nutrition Services for Medicare Beneficiaries. The role of nutrition in maintaining health in the nation's elderly: evaluating coverage of nutrition services for the Medicare population. Washington, DC: National Academy Press; 2000.
10. Pearson S, Inglis SC, McLennan SN, et al. Prolonged effects of a home-based intervention in patients with chronic illness. Arch Intern Med 2006;166:645–50.
11. Baker DW, Brown J, Chan KS, et al. A telephone survey to measure communication, education, self-management, and health status for patients with heart failure: the Improving Chronic Illness Care Evaluation (ICICE). J Card Fail 2005;11:36–42.
12. Krumholz HM, Baker DW, Ashton CM, et al. Evaluating quality of care for patients with heart failure. Circulation 2000;101:E122–40.
13. He J, Ogden LG, Bazzano LA, et al. Dietary sodium intake and incidence of congestive heart failure in overweight US men and women: first National Health and Nutrition Examination Survey Epidemiologic Follow-up Study. Arch Intern Med 2002;162:1619–24.
14. Opasich C, Rapezzi C, Lucci D, et al. Precipitating factors and decision-making processes of short-term worsening heart failure despite "optimal" treatment (from the IN-CHF Registry). Am J Cardiol 2001;88:382–7.
15. Opasich C, Febo O, Riccardi PG, et al. Concomitant factors of decompensation in chronic heart failure. Am J Cardiol 1996;78:354–7.
16. Dickstein K. ESC Guidelines for the diagnosis and treatment of acute and chronic heart failure 2008. Eur Heart J 2008;29(19):2388–442.
17. Witte KK, Clark AL, Cleland JG. Chronic heart failure and micronutrients. J Am Coll Cardiol 2001;37:1765–74.
18. Sole MJ, Jeejeebhoy KN. Conditioned nutritional requirements: therapeutic relevance to heart failure. Herz 2002;27:174–8.
19. Vivekananthan DP, Penn MS, Sapp SK, et al. Use of antioxidant vitamins for the prevention of cardiovascular disease: meta-analysis of randomised trials. Lancet 2003;361:2017–23.
20. Lonn E, Bosch J, Yusuf S, et al. Effects of long-term vitamin E supplementation on cardiovascular events and cancer: a randomized controlled trial. JAMA 2005;293:1338–47.
21. McQueen MJ, Lonn E, Gerstein HC, et al. The HOPE (Heart Outcomes Prevention Evaluation) Study and its consequences. Scand J Clin Lab Invest Suppl 2005;240:143–56.
22. Seligmann H, Halkin H, Rauchfleisch S, et al. Thiamine deficiency in patients with congestive heart failure receiving long-term furosemide therapy: a pilot study. Am J Med 1991;91:151–5.
23. Zenuk C, Healey J, Donnelly J, et al. Thiamine deficiency in congestive heart failure patients receiving long term furosemide therapy. Can J Clin Pharmacol 2003;10:184–8.
24. Brady JA, Rock CL, Horneffer MR. Thiamin status, diuretic medications, and the management of congestive heart failure. J Am Diet Assoc 1995;95:541–4.
25. Hanninen SA, Darling PB, Sole MJ, et al. The prevalence of thiamin deficiency in hospitalized patients

with congestive heart failure. J Am Coll Cardiol 2006; 47:354–61.

26. Shimon I, Almog S, Vered Z, et al. Improved left ventricular function after thiamine supplementation in patients with congestive heart failure receiving long-term furosemide therapy. Am J Med 1995;98:485–90.

27. Smithline HA. Thiamine for the treatment of acute decompensated heart failure. Am J Emerg Med 2007;25:124–6.

28. Keith ME, Walsh NA, Darling PB, et al. B-vitamin deficiency in hospitalized patients with heart failure. J Am Diet Assoc 2009;109:1406–10.

29. Vasan RS, Beiser A, D'Agostino RB, et al. Plasma homocysteine and risk for congestive heart failure in adults without prior myocardial infarction. JAMA 2003;289:1251–7.

30. Herrmann M, Muller S, Kindermann I, et al. Plasma B vitamins and their relation to the severity of chronic heart failure. Am J Clin Nutr 2007;85:117–23.

31. Li YC, Kong J, Wei M, et al. 1,25-Dihydroxyvitamin D(3) is a negative endocrine regulator of the renin-angiotensin system. J Clin Invest 2002;110:229–38.

32. O'Connell TD, Simpson RU. 1,25-Dihydroxyvitamin D3 regulation of myocardial growth and c-myc levels in the rat heart. Biochem Biophys Res Commun 1995;213:59–65.

33. Nibbelink KA, Tishkoff DX, Hershey SD, et al. 1,25(OH)2-vitamin D3 actions on cell proliferation, size, gene expression, and receptor localization, in the HL-1 cardiac myocyte. J Steroid Biochem Mol Biol 2007;103:533–7.

34. Boxer RS, Dauser DA, Walsh SJ, et al. The association between vitamin D and inflammation with the 6-minute walk and frailty in patients with heart failure. J Am Geriatr Soc 2008;56:454–61.

35. Boxer RS, Kenny AM, Cheruvu VK, et al. Serum 25-hydroxyvitamin D concentration is associated with functional capacity in older adults with heart failure. Am Heart J 2010;160(5):893–9.

36. Bischoff-Ferrari HA, Dietrich T, Orav EJ, et al. Higher 25-hydroxyvitamin D concentrations are associated with better lower-extremity function in both active and inactive persons aged > or =60 y. Am J Clin Nutr 2004;80:752–8.

37. Houston DK, Cesari M, Ferrucci L, et al. Association between vitamin D status and physical performance: the InCHIANTI study. J Gerontol A Biol Sci Med Sci 2007;62:440–6.

38. Visser M, Deeg DJ, Lips P. Low vitamin D and high parathyroid hormone levels as determinants of loss of muscle strength and muscle mass (sarcopenia): the Longitudinal Aging Study Amsterdam. J Clin Endocrinol Metab 2003;88:5766–72.

39. Liu W, Guo M, Ezzat S, et al. Vitamin D inhibits CEA-CAM1 to promote insulin/IGF-I receptor signaling without compromising anti-proliferative action. Lab Invest 2011;91(1):147–56.

40. Zittermann A, Schleithoff SS, Tenderich G, et al. Low vitamin D status: a contributing factor in the pathogenesis of congestive heart failure? J Am Coll Cardiol 2003;41:105–12.

41. Pilz S, Marz W, Wellnitz B, et al. Association of vitamin D deficiency with heart failure and sudden cardiac death in a large cross-sectional study of patients referred for coronary angiography. J Clin Endocrinol Metab 2008;93:3927–35.

42. Witham MD, Crighton LJ, Gillespie ND, et al. The effects of vitamin D supplementation on physical function and quality of life in older patients with heart failure: a randomized controlled trial. Circ Heart Fail 2010;3:195–201.

43. Schleithoff SS, Zittermann A, Tenderich G, et al. Vitamin D supplementation improves cytokine profiles in patients with congestive heart failure: a double-blind, randomized, placebo-controlled trial. Am J Clin Nutr 2006;83:754–9.

44. Rich MW, Beckham V, Wittenberg C, et al. A multidisciplinary intervention to prevent the readmission of elderly patients with congestive heart failure. N Engl J Med 1995;333:1190–5.

45. Bandura A. Human agency in social cognitive theory. Am Psychol 1989;44:1175–84.

46. Scotto CJ. The lived experience of adherence for patients with heart failure. J Cardiopulm Rehabil 2005;25:158–63.

47. Riegel B, Moser DK, Anker SD, et al. State of the science: promoting self-care in persons with heart failure: a scientific statement from the American Heart Association. Circulation 2009;120:1141–63.

48. Bodenheimer T, Lorig K, Holman H, et al. Patient self-management of chronic disease in primary care. JAMA 2002;288:2469–75.

49. Flynn KJ, Powell LH, Mendes de Leon CF, et al. Increasing self-management skills in heart failure patients: a pilot study. Congest Heart Fail 2005;11:297–302.

50. Powell LH, Calvin JE Jr, Mendes de Leon CF, et al. The Heart Failure Adherence and Retention Trial (HART): design and rationale. Am Heart J 2008;156:452–60.

51. Powell LH, Calvin JE Jr, Richardson D, et al. Self-management counseling in patients with heart failure: the heart failure adherence and retention randomized behavioral trial. JAMA 2010;304:1331–8.

52. Haynes RB, Yao X, Degani A, et al. Interventions to enhance medication adherence. Cochrane Database Syst Rev 2005;4:CD000011.

53. World Health Organization. Adherence to long-term therapies: evidence for action. Available at: http://www.who.int/chp/knowledge/publications/adherence_full_report.pdf.

54. O'connor CM, Whellan DJ, Lee KL, et al. Efficacy and safety of exercise training in patients with chronic

heart failure: HF-ACTION randomized controlled trial. JAMA 2009;301:1439–50.

55. Franciosa JA, Park M, Levine TB. Lack of correlation between exercise capacity and indexes of resting left ventricular performance in heart failure. Am J Cardiol 1981;47:33–9.

56. Pina IL, Fitzpatrick JT. Exercise and heart failure. A review. Chest 1996;110:1317–27.

57. Balady GJ, Arena R, Sietsema K, et al. Clinician's Guide to cardiopulmonary exercise testing in adults: a scientific statement from the American Heart Association. Circulation 2010;122:191–225.

58. Braunschweig F, Linde C, Adamson PB, et al. Continuous central haemodynamic measurements during the six-minute walk test and daily life in patients with chronic heart failure. Eur J Heart Fail 2009;11:594–601.

59. Clark AL, Poole-Wilson PA, Coats AJ. Exercise limitation in chronic heart failure: central role of the periphery. J Am Coll Cardiol 1996;28:1092–102.

60. Franciosa JA, Baker BJ, Seth L. Pulmonary versus systemic hemodynamics in determining exercise capacity of patients with chronic left ventricular failure. Am Heart J 1985;110:807–13.

61. Mancini DM, Eisen H, Kussmaul W, et al. Value of peak exercise oxygen consumption for optimal timing of cardiac transplantation in ambulatory patients with heart failure. Circulation 1991;83:778–86.

62. Convertino VA, Goldwater DJ, Sandler H. Bedrest-induced peak VO2 reduction associated with age, gender, and aerobic capacity. Aviat Space Environ Med 1986;57:17–22.

63. Convertino VA. Cardiovascular consequences of bed rest: effect on maximal oxygen uptake. Med Sci Sports Exerc 1997;29:191–6.

64. Ades PA, Pashkow FJ, Fletcher G, et al. A controlled trial of cardiac rehabilitation in the home setting using electrocardiographic and voice transtelephonic monitoring. Am Heart J 2000;139:543–8.

65. Belardinelli R, Scocco V, Mazzanti M, et al. Effects of aerobic training in patients with moderate chronic heart failure. G Ital Cardiol 1992;22:919–30 [in Italian].

66. Dubach P, Myers J, Dziekan G, et al. Effect of high intensity exercise training on central hemodynamic responses to exercise in men with reduced left ventricular function. J Am Coll Cardiol 1997;29:1591–8.

67. Giannuzzi P, Temporelli PL, Corra U, et al. Antiremodeling effect of long-term exercise training in patients with stable chronic heart failure: results of the Exercise in Left Ventricular Dysfunction and Chronic Heart Failure (ELVD-CHF) Trial. Circulation 2003;108:554–9.

68. Keteyian SJ. Exercise rehabilitation in chronic heart failure. Coron Artery Dis 2006;17:233–7.

69. Hambrecht R, Wolf A, Gielen S, et al. Effect of exercise on coronary endothelial function in patients with coronary artery disease. N Engl J Med 2000;342:454–60.

70. Flynn KE, Pina IL, Whellan DJ, et al. Effects of exercise training on health status in patients with chronic heart failure: HF-ACTION randomized controlled trial. JAMA 2009;301:1451–9.

71. Fletcher GF, Balady GJ, Amsterdam EA, et al. Exercise standards for testing and training: a statement for healthcare professionals from the American Heart Association. Circulation 2001;104:1694–740.

72. World Health Organization. Preparation and use of food-based dietary guidelines. Report of a joint FAO/WHO consultation. (WHO Technical Report Series, No. 880). Geneva, 1998.

73. World Health Organization. Food based dietary guidelines in the WHO European region. (Report EUR/03/5045414/E79832). Nutrition and Food Security Programme, WHO Regional Office for Europe Copenhagen. 2003.

74. World Health Organization. Keep fit for life: Meeting the nutritional needs of older persons. Geneva, 2002.

75. Institute of Medicine, Food and Nutrition Board. Dietary Reference. Intakes: The Essential Reference for Dietary Planning and Assessment. National Academy of Sciences. Washington DC: National Academy Press; 2006.

76. US Department of Agriculture and US Department of Health and Human Services. Report of the 2005 Dietary Guidelines Advisory Committee. Washington DC, 2005.

77. National Heart, Lung, and Blood Institute. The DASH Eating Plan. National Institutes of Health, US Department of Health and Human Services, Bethesda, MD, 2006.

78. National Heart, Lung, and Blood Institute. Your Guide to Lowering Your Cholesterol with TLC (Therapeutic Lifestyle Changes). National Institutes of Health, US Department of Health and Human Services, Bethesda, MD, 2006.

79. Tangalos EG. Congestive heart failure. Nutrition management for older adults. Nutrition Screening Initiative, American Dietetic Association, Chicago, and American Academy of Family Physicians. Washington, DC, 2002.

End-Point Selection for Acute Heart Failure Trials

Larry A. Allen, MD, MHS*

KEYWORDS

- End points • Acute heart failure syndromes
- Acute decompensated heart failure
- Randomized controlled trial design

Acute heart failure (AHF) is a syndrome character-ized by new or worsening signs or symptoms of heart failure leading to hospitalization. AHF is responsible for 3.7 million heart failure–related hospitalizations in the United States each year, 1.1 million with a primary diagnosis of heart failure.[1] In stark contrast to significant therapeutic ad-vances in the care of patients with stable chronic heart failure and reduced left ventricular ejection fraction (LVEF),[2–4] trials in AHF have met with mini-mal success.[5,6] Faced with a variety of challenges inherent to the study of AHF—varied etiology, high comorbidity, poorly understood precipitants, a short time horizon for the application of many therapies, and a lack of successful therapeutic development examples to model—there has been little consensus in the research or regulatory community about a variety of aspects of clinical trial design in AHF, including end-point selection.

To advance the field of AHF therapy, there is a need to develop and promote end-point measures that encompass the totality of potential therapeutic benefits in AHF patients, including sustained relief of symptoms, reduced length of stay, decreased rehospitalization, and prolonged survival. Ulti-mately, for one therapeutic approach to be consid-ered superior to another, it must make patients live longer, make patients feel better, or save resources without adversely affecting these 2 aims. To reach this goal, greater standardization of end points across studies is needed for therapies to be easily compared and prioritized by patients, clinicians, and payers. In addition, better validated surrogates for both efficacy and safety are needed to help speed the development of new agents by reliably recognizing efficacy and safety issues earlier in the development process. Therefore, this review aims to build on prior reviews of this topic[7–10] by creating a framework of clinical and statistical concerns for end-point design, summarizing end points used in recent and ongoing AHF studies, describing changes to the current regulatory envi-ronment for the approval of AHF therapies, and suggesting options for the development of more robust end points moving forward.

A FRAMEWORK FOR END-POINT DESIGN IN AHF

End points in trials of medical therapies are specific, identifiable, downstream events or changes in a patient's condition. Ideal end points should be unambiguous, consistent, easy to obtain, inexpen-sive to measure, sensitive to the processes of care that they are designed to reflect, and simple to understand. Because AHF is highly symptomatic, affects multiple organ systems, is often lethal, and garners a large proportion of medical resources, a wide range of end-point options are available.

Yet AHF end-point design is far less developed than for other cardiovascular entities. For nearly 20 years, trials of neurohormonal antagonists and

Disclosures/Funding support: Dr Allen is funded by a Scientist Development Award from the American Heart Association, and has served as a consultant for Amgen and the Robert Wood Johnson Foundation.
Colorado Cardiovascular Outcomes Research Consortium and the Section of Advanced Heart Failure, Division of Cardiology, Department of Medicine, University of Colorado Denver, Anschutz Medical Campus, 12631 East 17th Avenue, Academic Office 1, Mailstop B130, PO Box 6511, Aurora, CO 80045, USA
* Academic Office 1, 12631 East 17th Avenue, Mailstop B130, PO Box 6511, Aurora, CO 80045.
E-mail address: larry.allen@ucdenver.edu

Heart Failure Clin 7 (2011) 481–495
doi:10.1016/j.hfc.2011.06.007
1551-7136/11/$ – see front matter © 2011 Elsevier Inc. All rights reserved.

heartfailure.theclinics.com

cardiac resynchronization therapy in patients with chronic systolic heart failure have demonstrated improvements in mortality and hospitalization, with relatively good surrogate markers of therapeutic efficacy captured through measures of ventricular remodeling (ie, left ventricular volumes). Similarly, the field of acute coronary syndromes has benefited from broad consensus around major cardiovascular events as a combined primary end point for drug development since the thrombolytic era. AHF has not followed these examples for several reasons. It is helpful to consider some of the unique clinical and statistical issues that have plagued AHF end-point development.

Foremost, the pathophysiology of AHF remains poorly understood. Because AHF is marked by the common symptoms of dyspnea and fatigue prompting urgent medical attention, these patients have often been lumped together for recruitment into AHF trials. It is becoming increasingly recognized that AHF captures a heterogeneous group of patients not only with respect to LVEF but also in terms of diastology, systemic vasoreactivity, right heart function, pulmonary hypertension, and cardiorenal interactions. Furthermore, there has clearly been an overemphasis of the role of fluid retention in the pathogenesis of AHF. A wide variety of therapies focused on volume control—loop diuretic dosing schemes,[11] adenosine receptor antagonists,[12] vasopressin receptor antagonists,[13,14] telemonitoring of daily weights,[15] implantable hemodynamic monitors,[16] and ultrafiltration[17]—have generally failed to show clinically significant improvements in patient-centered outcomes. In combination with data showing that a minority of patients gain significant weight proceeding an episode of AHF,[18] in hindsight these results are not surprising. Moreover, if we are to move away from volume status as the dominant paradigm in therapeutic target, end points measuring fluid loss, weight change, edema, and hemodynamic measures should also take a back seat. Greater efforts are being made to match particular therapies to groups of patients for which the mechanism of action is a prominent aspect of the AHF presentation, but these efforts are in their infancy.[19] Improving our understanding of specific pathophysiology, precipitants, and manifestations of AHF is necessary in the selection of relevant response variables.

Further complicating AHF end-point selection is the prominent role of noncardiovascular disease in patients presenting with AHF. Not only are the causes of AHF varied, but there is a complex overlay of comorbidity that affects the initial presentation, the response to therapy, and subsequent outcomes. Intermediate-term mortality and hospitalization have been held up as clinically important end points. However, among patients with a median age of 75 years who also have rates of diabetes, lung disease, and vascular disease exceeding 30%, much of the morbidity and mortality that can be measured is unlikely to be affected by AHF-specific therapy. Among Medicare beneficiaries who are readmitted within 30 days of a primary discharge diagnosis of heart failure, only 37% of those readmissions are again given a primary diagnosis of heart failure.[20] This finding has important implications for AHF trial design, including the selection of disease-specific end points.[21]

The acute nature of AHF poses a challenge as well. Unlike neurohormonal antagonist therapy, which is taken for years and for which trials collect end-point data for years, AHF therapies are often used for only hours to days. In addition, it is uncertain as to the extent to which short-term AHF therapies given during an index hospitalization can affect postdischarge mortality. In order for a short-term AHF therapy to affect mortality rates it would need to (1) significantly diminish in-hospital mortality, (2) alter the fundamental natural history of the AHF syndrome in a way that leads to a reduction in subsequent clinical events, or (3) facilitate the introduction or up-titration of chronic heart failure therapies known to improve survival. For example, acute reperfusion therapy for myocardial infarction conveys a long-term survival benefit by arresting the central pathophysiological mechanism, with subsequent prevention of disease progression. Whether such a paradigm can be translated to AHF therapies is unknown, given that no overarching fundamental mechanism has been identified for this heterogeneous family of disorders.

Serial failures of several AHF trials have deprived the field of a standard model from which to build on. Consequently, AHF end-point selection for clinical trials represents a constantly shifting landscape. Initial therapies for AHF such as loop diuretics were accepted into practice largely on pharmacokinetic and pharmacodynamic data supplemented with anecdotal clinical experience. Milrinone was approved for AHF by the United States Food and Drug Administration (FDA) in 1988 based primarily on its hemodynamic effects. The next agent approved by the FDA specifically for use in AHF was nesiritide in 2001, based on short-term improvements in both hemodynamics and patient-reported dyspnea within the first 24 hours. Subsequently, there have been substantial concerns raised about the safety and efficacy of both milrinone[22] and nesiritide,[23–26] which led to increased skepticism about these prior end points. As a result, multiple novel therapies for AHF have been tested in a variety of clinical trials in the last decade, almost all of which used differing end points and which have resulted in a variety of interpretations (**Table 1**).[27]

It is within this complicated landscape that we consider end-point selection for AHF trials. As the various types of end points that can be measured in clinical trials of AHF are reviewed, it is helpful to keep in mind the advantages and disadvantages of each end point and possible combinations as they relate to the aforementioned considerations.

PATIENT-CENTERED CLINICAL END POINTS

In general, the FDA mandates that for a therapy to be approved it has to make patients feel better and/or live longer.[28] Consequently, pivotal phase 3 trials of new therapies must demonstrate clinically relevant improvement in a patient-centered clinical end point (as distinct from a surrogate end point) in order to justify regulatory approval and clinical use.

Vital Status

Survival is an important end point to consider in any clinical syndrome associated with substantial risk of death (eg, AHF), and has been the gold standard for trials. Vital status is objective and easy to assess. Vital status can be obtained through a variety of mechanisms, ensuring complete capture. Prolonging survival is also the number-one priority for most patients with AHF.[29]

Despite its obvious appeal as an end point for AHF trials, mortality has not been used as the sole primary end point in any large AHF trials, for good reason. Although AHF is a highly morbid condition with in-hospital mortality rates on the order of 4% to 7% and 30-day mortality rates of approximately 11%,[1] trial designs have not targeted mortality alone because of the high prevalence of comorbidities and the recurrent failure of short-term AHF therapies to positively influence survival.

Controversy also exists about whether it is preferable to measure all-cause or disease-specific mortality.[21] All-cause mortality has the advantage of a higher overall event rate than disease-specific mortality, as well as requiring no adjudication as to cause of death. However, all-cause mortality will include events that are unlikely to be responsive to the therapy being tested, which will tend to diminish the overall power of the analysis through greater standard error. Disease-specific event rates related to the specific mechanism of action of the therapy (eg, sudden death in defibrillator trials) are much more likely to demonstrate a treatment effect, assuming that the mechanism of action of the therapy is reasonably well understood and the end point can be accurately classified. It should be noted that therapies that reduce one mode of death may inadvertently be associated with increases in another (eg, arrhythmic death vs nonarrhythmic death with the implantation of defibrillators for heart failure immediately after myocardial infarction),[30] and thus even if a disease-specific cause of death is chosen, ideally all-cause mortality would also be reported. The use of disease-specific event rates generally necessitates the use of clinical adjudication of cause of death. A significant portion of misclassification is common in the collection of cause of death (death certificates are notoriously inaccurate[31]), which can be at least partially corrected with data audits and blinded adjudication.[32] Data from heart failure trials among patients with reduced LVEF have found that most postdischarge deaths are cardiovascular in nature.[33,34] Although the relatively older age and higher degree of comorbidity among patients with heart failure and normal LVEF produces a higher proportion of noncardiovascular mortality, the majority of deaths remain cardiovascular in nature.[35,36] Therefore, the use of all-cause mortality may be most advantageous in the AHF population, despite recommendations otherwise.[21]

Health Status

Symptoms, functional status, and quality of life are primary concerns for patients. Nearly half of patients with symptomatic heart failure would make health-care decisions that improve their quality of life at the expense of its quantity.[29,37,38] AHF in particular is related to health status, with worsening symptoms of fatigue, shortness of breath, and edema defining the syndrome. These symptoms, in turn, can limit physical and social activities and impair emotional functioning. The degree to which symptoms and functional limitations differ from patients' expectations for their health determines how much worse their quality of life will be. As such, improvements in health status represent a central goal of AHF therapy.

Although survival and health status both represent critical patient-centered outcomes, health status measures have traditionally been considered a "softer" end point, because they represent subjective reports from patients. Nevertheless, the reproducibility and sensitivity to clinical change of standardized questionnaires is better than many other modalities of quantifying patients' function.[39]

In clinical research studies, there are several methods for quantifying the impact of the disease on patients' health status. An important consideration is whether generic health status measures or

Table 1
Selected large AHF trials and their end points

Acronym	Year of Publication	Intervention	Primary End Point(s)	Main Secondary End Points	Comments
VMAC[53]	2002	Nesiritide infusion 48 h vs nitroglycerine infusion vs placebo	Coprimary: 1. Δ PCWP at 3 h 2. Δ dyspnea (Likert) at 3 h	PCWP at 24 h, dyspnea at 24 and 48 h, global clinical status	Approved based on improvement in primary end points. Tertiary end points unchanged: 48-h hypotension; 30-d mortality, myocardial infarction, readmission, and renal dysfunction; 6-mo mortality (but not powered for these). ASCEND-HF subsequently showed no significant difference (below)
OPTIME[22]	2002	Milrinone infusion 48 h vs placebo	Cumulative days of hospitalization for cardiovascular cause or days dead within 60 d following randomization	Proportion of cases failing therapy due to adverse events or worsening heart failure (sustained SBP <80 mm Hg, myocardial ischemia, arrhythmias, persistent CHF, inadequate diuresis, organ hypoperfusion), heart failure score, global health (VAS)	Safety end points trended against milrinone
VERITAS[52]	2007	Tezosentan infusion 24–72 h vs placebo	Coprimary: 1. Δ dyspnea (at 3, 6, and 24 h using VAS 0–100) over 24 h (area under the curve) 2. Death or worsening heart failure (pulmonary edema, shock, new or ↑ IV therapy, mechanical cardiac or pulmonary support, renal replacement therapy) at 7 d	Death or major cardiovascular events at 30 d; improved hemodynamic measures over 24 h; length of stay; days hospitalized within 30 d; 6-mo mortality	All primary and secondary end points were not significantly affected by treatment

SURVIVE[78]	2007	Levosimendan infusion vs dobutamine infusion as long as clinically indicated in AHF patients requiring inotropic support	All-cause mortality at 180 d	All-cause mortality at 31 d; days alive or out of hospital at 180 d; cardiovascular mortality at 180 d; change in BNP level at 24 h; dyspnea at 24 h; patient-assessed global assessment at 24 h	Only difference seen was in BNP levels. Concerns over use of an appropriate comparator therapy
REVIVE-2[68]	Presented 2005	Levosimendan infusion vs placebo in hemodynamically stable AHF patients	Composite of clinical signs and symptoms of heart failure over 5 d expressed as 3-stage end point: 1. Better (moderately or markedly improved global assessment at 6 h, 24 h, and 5 d with no worsening) 2. Same 3. Worse (death from any cause, persistent or worsening heart failure requiring intravenous diuretics, vasodilators, or inotropes at any time; or moderately or markedly worse patient global assessment at 6 h, 24 h, or 5 d)	Change in BNP, hypotension, ventricular tachycardia, atrial fibrillation; mortality at 90 d	The primary end point was improved, as was BNP; however, concerns about strong trends in increased hypotension, arrhythmia, and 90-day mortality led FDA not to approve the drug

(continued on next page)

Table 1
(continued)

Acronym	Year of Publication	Intervention	Primary End Point(s)	Main Secondary End Points	Comments
EVEREST[13,14]	2007	Tolvaptan oral vs placebo up to 112 wk	Short-term composite at day 7 or hospital discharge: 1. Δ global clinical status (VAS), and 2. Δ body weight Long-term dual safety end points, time-to-event: 1. All-cause mortality (superiority and noninferiority) 2. Cardiovascular death or heart failure hospitalization (superiority only)	Composite components in isolation at days 1 and 7 or discharge; dyspnea at day 1; peripheral edema at day 7 or discharge; Kansas City Cardiomyopathy Questionnaire at 1 wk and 6 mo; body weight; changes in serum sodium	Atypical AHF trial, in that therapy was continued indefinitely. Long-term clinical measures were designed as the main safety end point, but failure to improve these despite small gains in global clinical status and body weight led to questions about clinical efficacy. The FDA approved tolvaptan only for a hyponatremia indication, not AHF
ASCEND-HF[23,24]	Presented 2011	Nesiritide infusion vs placebo	Coprimary: 1. Composite of all-cause mortality and heart failure rehospitalization through 30 d 2. Dyspnea at 6 and 24 h	Overall well-being (Likert) 6 and 24 h; days alive and outside of hospital within 30 d	Primary end point

Trial	Status	Intervention	Primary End Point	Secondary	Comments
PROTECT[12]	2010	Rolofylline infusion vs placebo	Composite of clinical signs and symptoms of heart failure over 7 d expressed as 3-stage end point: 1. Better (moderately or markedly improved global assessment at 24 and 48 h with no worsening) 2. Same 3. Worse (death from any cause, persistent or worsening heart failure through day 7, or creatinine increase ≥0.3 mg/dL at 7 and 14 d)	Safety; within trial costs	No evidence of efficacy; increased neurologic events. Phase 2 development study involved numerous end points to guide post hoc phase 3 end-point selection[79]
RELAX-AHF[81]	Enrolling	Relaxin infusion for 48 h vs placebo	Signs and symptoms of acute heart failure	Renal function	Phase 2 trial explored multiple potential end points,[82] leading to end-point selection for this study

Abbreviations: Δ, changed; ASCEND-HF, Acute Study of Clinical Effectiveness of Nesiritide in Decompensated Heart Failure; BNP, brain natriuretic peptide; CHF, congestive heart failure; EVEREST, Efficacy of Vasopressin Antagonism in Heart Failure Outcome Study with Tolvaptan; FDA, Food and Drug Administration; IV, intravenous; MLwHF, Minnesota Living with Heart Failure questionnaire; mm Hg, millimeters mercury; OPTIME, Outcomes of a Prospective Trial of Intravenous Milrinone for Exacerbations of Chronic Heart Failure; PCWP, post-capillary wedge pressure; PROTECT, Placebo-Controlled Randomized Study of the Selective A₁ Adenosine Receptor Antagonist Rolofylline for Patients Hospitalized with Acute Decompensated Heart Failure and Volume Overload to Assess Treatment Effect on Congestion and Renal Function; RELAX-AHF, Efficacy and Safety of Relaxin for the Treatment of Acute Heart Failure; REVIVE-2, Second Randomized Multicenter Evaluation of Intravenous Levosimendan Efficacy; SBP, systolic blood pressure; SURVIVE, Survival of Patients with Acute Heart Failure in Need of Intravenous Inotropic Support; VAS, visual analog scale; VERITAS, Value of Endothelin Receptor Inhibition with Tezosentan in Acute Heart Failure Study; VMAC, Vasodilation in the Management of Acute CHF.

Modified from Allen LA, Hernandez AF, O'Connor CM, et al. End points for clinical trials in acute heart failure syndromes. J Am Coll Cardiol 2009;53(24):2252; with permission.

a disease-specific measure should be used. Generic instruments quantify the overall health of patients, including heart failure and all other comorbidities that patients may have. Common examples include the EuroQol (EQ-5D),[40] the Health Utilities Index (HUI),[41] and the 12- or 36-item short-form questionnaires (SF-12 or SF-36).[42] While the advantage of these measures is that they can permit comparisons between heart failure treatments and treatments for other diseases on a common scale as well as map to health utilities, they are much less sensitive to important clinical changes than disease-specific measures.[43,44]

Several disease-specific health status measures have been developed for patients with heart failure. The two most commonly used disease-specific health status instruments are the Minnesota Living with Heart Failure Questionnaire (MLwHF)[45] and the Kansas City Cardiomyopathy Questionnaire (KCCQ).[43] The KCCQ has been shown to be more sensitive to changes in clinical status than EuroQol (EQ-5D), SF-12, 6-minute walk test, and New York Heart Association (NYHA) functional classification.[46] Although these questionnaires were designed to quantify patient health status, they have also been associated with prognosis for survival and costs.[47–51] Yet despite the psychometric and prognostic validity of the MLwHF and KCCQ, they have seldom been used in AHF trials,[39] due in part to the development of these instruments in the chronic stable heart failure population. KCCQ questions ask about how heart failure has affected a patient "over the past 2 weeks," when symptoms during an episode of AHF may change rapidly over hours to days. Single-item measures of patient-reported global health status (general well-being) have been the standard for AHF trials.[13] However, such single-item measures are unlikely to perform as well as more complex questionnaires designed to monitor multiple domains of health status.

Targeted patient-reported symptom measures, primarily dyspnea, have been commonly used as primary end points in large AHF trials over the past decade, either alone or in combination with other measures. Many contemporary phase 3 AHF trials have monitored some measure of short-term changes in dyspnea.[17,23,24,52,53] Dyspnea is the most common presenting symptom for patients with AHF, and hospital discharge is often dictated by resolution in dyspnea. Despite the ascendance of dyspnea as a key measure of efficacy in AHF trials over the past decade, there are significant issues regarding dyspnea as an end point. No validated instrument for dyspnea assessment currently exists that is accurate, reliable, reproducible between observers, and sensitive to important changes in dyspnea.[54] This shortcoming has led to the use of an assortment of poorly validated instruments for assessing dyspnea, including Likert scales, visual analog scales, and more complicated measures.[54–56] Furthermore, patterns of dyspnea resolution appear to be significantly affected by choice of response instrument.[57] Also problematic for the use of dyspnea as a primary end point is the possibility of relatively rapid improvement irrespective of therapy for AHF. In the placebo arms of recent AHF studies, substantial relief of dyspnea is seen within 24 to 48 hours using standard therapy alone. Studies requiring a more objective measure of disease severity for patient enrollment (such as natriuretic peptide levels) have shown less degree of dyspnea improvement in the placebo group, suggesting that more severely ill patients may have greater degrees of unresolved dyspnea that could serve as a target for dyspnea-reducing therapy.[12] In order for an incremental improvement in dyspnea to be considered a significant therapeutic advance, it would need to be relatively rapid, of substantial magnitude, and sustained beyond the initial few hours of therapy.

Changes in the 4-tier NYHA functional classification, developed in 1928 and last revised 17 years ago, have frequently been used as a measure of improved status in AHF studies.[58] However, the NYHA classification suffers from several critical limitations. First, it reflects patients' health status from physicians' perspectives and not from patients themselves. Second, its validity and reproducibility have been questioned.[59,60]

Regardless of the instrument used, health status measures must be prospectively obtained on multiple occasions via direct input from the patient. More frequent collection over time has obvious advantages in terms of characterizing patients' overall experience, but this requires ongoing solicitation. Missing health status assessments, like any missing data, can severely undermine the internal validity of the analysis. In addition to vigilant efforts to limit missing data, predefined methods to account for loss to follow-up and incorporation of deaths is critical to accurate presentation and interpretation of health status findings.

RESOURCE USE AND COST

Cost represents the third major category of end points that relate to the value of AHF therapies. With growing pressure to control health care expenditures, economic end points are likely to become increasingly collected and reported. However, without considering the totality of a therapy, including its impact on downstream outcomes and safety, cost analyses can lead to false estimates of savings and potentially undermine valuable care options.[61] Therefore, the goal must be to compare the relative value (efficiency) of AHF therapy options, by combining total costs with a comprehensive assessment of benefits and risks. The National Institute for Health and Clinical Excellence (NICE), a special authority of the National Health Service (NHS) in England and Wales, effectively requires cost and utility data to be collected in the drug-development process. Although Americans have generally shown less tolerance for such centralized regulation, there is growing interest in the United States in reducing health care use though free choice in response to pricing mechanisms.[62]

To perform cost-effectiveness analyses of new therapies for AHF, ideally a wide range of end points need to be prospectively collected during the conduct of large AHF trials, which would include both medical and nonmedical costs. In addition, which resources are included in the end point of cost are highly dependent on the perspective chosen, that is, the patient versus the health system versus the insurance payor versus society at large. A full discussion of end points for cost-effectiveness analyses in AHF is beyond the scope of this review, other than to say that attention to prospective collection of cost measures is warranted in phase 3 AHF trials.

HYBRID CLINICAL MEASURES
Hospitalization and Readmission

Much of the burden of heart failure is the result of inpatient care. Hospitalization and readmission for AHF is associated with severe symptoms, diminished quality of life, and poor postdischarge prognosis. Approximately 70% of total direct costs for heart failure are attributable to inpatient care.[63] For patients hospitalized with AHF, both the length of stay for the index hospitalization (median of 6 days in the United States) and the risk of readmission (approximately 20% at 30 days) are substantial. Thus, addressing the morbidity of AHF by limiting length of stay and reducing readmission is an obvious objective in AHF.

Unlike mortality end points, hospitalization end points may be substantially affected by social preferences and regional differences in practice patterns. For example, length of stay for AHF in European counties is significantly longer than in the United States (see the article by Mona Fiuzat and Robert M. Califf, on regional differences elsewhere in this issue).[64,65] In addition, the increased use of "short stay" holding units in emergency departments and the use of intravenous medications in heart failure clinics can confound the definition of hospitalization, a practice that may increase as financial incentives within the Affordable Care Act designed to reduce readmissions take effect. Decisions about what type of hospitalization to measure (ie, all-cause vs cardiovascular vs heart failure related) generally reflect the same concerns that are already discussed for all-cause versus disease-specific mortality.[66]

Methods for quantifying the burden of hospitalization in AHF have varied between studies. Traditional "time-to-event" analyses using Cox proportional hazards models, which have become standard in chronic heart failure trials, may be less relevant when the follow-up period is relatively short or when multiple or prolonged hospitalizations are common. In addition, the end point of "readmission" is paradoxically related to the length of stay of the index hospitalization, because patients with prolonged index hospitalizations have less time at risk for rehospitalization.[23,24] Similarly, hospitalization must be considered in the context of overall mortality, because patients who do not survive are not at risk for rehospitalization. A composite of death or heart failure hospitalization has been used as the coprimary end point for the two largest AHF trials completed to date, the EVEREST and ASCEND-HF studies.[14,23,24]

Another approach that may more completely capture the burden of mortality and hospitalization during the follow-up period is the end point of "days alive and out of the hospital."[22,67] The theoretical advantage of this end point is that it combines mortality, length of stay of the index hospitalization, and the burden of subsequent hospitalizations into a single end point. However, when index length of stay is especially long (which may be of particular concern in studies enrolling a majority of patients outside North America), it may lead to decreased power.

Worsening Heart Failure/Need for Rescue Therapy

Recognition that commonly used short-term dyspnea end points and longer-term hospitalization end points neglect the critical time between initial stabilization and eventual hospital discharge has led to the development of "worsening heart failure" during therapy as an outcome measure in AHF. Although there is no consensus definition of worsening heart failure, typically it is defined as either failure to improve (persistent or worsening signs and symptoms of heart failure despite therapy) and/or need to intensify therapy (increased diuretic dose, initiation of intravenous vasoactive agents, or implementation of mechanical cardiac or ventilatory support). Multiple recent trials have utilized worsening heart failure end points as either a component of the primary end point or an important secondary end point,[12,52,68] but their validity as a patient-centered clinical end point remains in question.[69]

Renal Function

AHF is commonly accompanied by worsening renal function, sometimes referred to as the cardiorenal syndrome.[70] Worsening renal function, as defined by increasing serum creatinine, has been shown to be a powerful predictor of adverse outcomes in AHF,[71] and adenosine antagonist trials have targeted preservation of renal function as a therapeutic goal in AHF syndromes.[12] End-stage renal disease requiring renal replacement therapy has obvious implications for mortality, quality of life, and cost; however, changes in serum creatinine as little 0.3 mg/dL (the common definition of cardiorenal syndrome) may not have obvious clinical relevance to patients. As such, measures of renal function, although sometimes considered clinical end points and safety end points, under most circumstances should be considered a surrogate end point (see later discussion).

SURROGATES

Surrogate end points are response variables used to provide an indirect measurement of effect in situations where direct measurement of clinical effect is not feasible or practical.[72] To be valid, a surrogate end point should meet clearly defined criteria: (1) the surrogate must be in the causal pathway from the intervention to the clinically relevant outcome, as reflected by a strong association between the surrogate and the target; and (2) there must be no important effects of the intervention on the outcome which are not mediated through or captured by the surrogate.[73] Because it is challenging to establish that these criteria are met, surrogate measures are generally not accepted as proof of efficacy but rather as a signal of effect. Recent concerns about well-established surrogate end points (cholesterol, blood pressure, and glucose reduction) support this premise.[74,75] Nevertheless, surrogate outcomes continue to have an important role in the development of new therapies, because they often provide a more immediate manifestation of effect and typically allow for shorter and smaller trials in early phase development. Consequently, early-phase clinical studies designed to provide "proof of concept" or to select dosing for larger studies typically employ surrogate end points.

Unfortunately, the history of drug development in AHF has been marked by the frequent failure of surrogate end points to accurately predict clinical outcomes in larger efficacy trials. Until just a few years ago, changes in hemodynamics had been the primary focus of therapies for AHF. However, despite the short-term hemodynamic benefits of nesiritide and milrinone, the failure of these agents to positively influence patient-centered outcomes has significantly undermined our reliance on filling pressures and cardiac output as markers of clinical benefit. Similarly, decrease in body weight and net fluid loss have not corresponded with dyspnea or global health status measures.[13,17] Biomarkers, particularly the natriuretic peptides but also measures of acute kidney injury, inflammation, and troponins, have recently been promoted as surrogates for AHF studies.[76,77] However, their utility is also in question, particularly as trials of dobutamine and levosimendan have decreased natriuretic peptides without a corresponding improvement in overall clinical outcomes.[68,78] A thorough review of biomarkers as surrogate end points in heart failure trials by G. Michael Felker is included elsewhere in this issue.

SAFETY END POINTS

Given the history of drug development in AHF, the overall safety profile of new AHF therapies is an issue of significant concern. In particular, when the focus of a therapy is short-term symptom relief, establishing that this does not occur at the expense of longer-term safety is critical. Evaluation of safety for new therapies should be guided by an understanding of drug mechanism as well as by signals from earlier clinical study (eg, renal dysfunction with nesiritide, ischemia with inotropic agents). This approach requires testing specific safety hypotheses with the appropriate sample size that reasonably balances the desire to limit the risk for potential postapproval adverse events with the need for efficient pathways for evaluating new therapies. Often safety events are rare enough or occur over such long periods that they can only be determined through postmarketing phase 4 surveillance. Ultimately, the degree of risk that must be "ruled out" to declare a treatment "safe" should be related to the degree and type of benefit (ie, a drug that improves short-term symptoms only may be held to a higher standard of safety than one with more substantive clinical benefits).

COMPOSITE AND RANKED END POINTS

Given challenges in obtaining adequate power to capture important differences in patients' experience with AHF, substantial interest exists for combining end points to measure the impact of interventions on the various domains of possible benefit. One method for addressing these issues is the use of multiple primary end points. Using more than one primary end point requires appropriate adjustment for multiple statistical comparisons. Typically this takes the form of allocating the alpha (the potential for type I error) between the various end points. For example, ASCEND-HF used coprimary end points of (1) death or heart failure hospitalization at 180 days (alpha = 0.045) and (2) dyspnea assessment at 6 and 24 hours (alpha = 0.005).[23,24] In early phase development, some have argued that strict adjustments for multiple comparisons are not necessary during hypothesis generation, but this obviously increases the change of spurious findings, as was seen with the rolofylline development program.[12,79]

Distinct from the use of multiple primary end points, composite end points attempt to combine the various aspects of the AHF syndrome into a single integrated measure. Composite measures may be necessary to incorporate competing events (eg, death into measures of health status or hospitalization), but ranked end points may be a better way of doing so (see later discussion). Statistically, the use of composites increases the total event rate and therefore may increase statistical power. Importantly, however, composite end points only increase statistical power if the intervention has an effect on multiple aspects of the composite.

Another alternative to these composite end points are hierarchical end points based on ranking of events, sometimes termed the "global rank approach." In this type of scheme, all patients participating in a clinical trial are ranked based on a prespecified hierarchy of events. For example, time to death would be ranked at the bottom, then stroke, then hospitalization, then changes in health status, and so forth. The primary analysis in this type of analysis is the nonparametric comparison of the ranks. One advantage of this type of end point is that it "weighs" the components of the clinical experience in a way that is generally congruent with clinical judgment and patient-perceived value. A comprehensive review of this topic has been previously published.[10]

REGULATORY ISSUES

Regulatory requirements for approval of new drugs for AHF have evolved rapidly over the past decade in response to many of the AHF trial failures. At present, harmonization of regulatory agencies is lacking, often resulting in AHF studies with multiple primary end points designed to meet divergent regulatory requirements. This uncertainty as to how to interpret the evidence has led to AHF therapies that are approved by for use in the United States but not in Europe (nesiritide), and conversely drugs approved for use in Europe but not in the United States (levosimendan).

Furthermore, the FDA has recently directed that individual study populations for clinical trials require a unique patient-reported outcome measure to quantify health status.[80] The theory is that each study population, and disease state, has unique clinical issues, from patients' perspectives, that render more standard measures irrelevant. In AHF there is no empirical evidence to support this contention or guide specific development. Moreover, to be acceptable to the FDA for approval, the measure must meet the standard psychometric properties of validity, reliability, responsiveness, and interpretability. Demonstrating these properties requires testing, expense, and time. This policy provides a substantial disincentive for the pharmaceutical and device industry to measure health status in their clinical trials, at a time when such measures appear to be emerging as a reasonable clinical end point for phase 3 AHF trials.

KEY CONSIDERATIONS FOR FUTURE END-POINT DESIGN

The aforementioned considerations help define general principles to guide future AHF end-point selection. First and foremost, phase 3 trials of AHF therapies must focus on measures of clinical importance assessed over a reasonable duration. Thus, treatments and trials designed to improve these outcomes should be a primary goal of research and development in AHF. While symptom relief remains an important goal of therapy, symptomatic improvement (in the absence of other clinical benefits) must be rapid, substantial, and sustained beyond the initial hours of treatment to be considered a significant therapeutic advance over usual care. As with all drug development, improved methods for postmarketing safety surveillance using valid end points are needed, but are even more important for therapies that appear to produce short-term symptomatic benefit. Moving forward, standardization and validation of end-point measures is critical, particularly as our understanding of the pathophysiology of AHF becomes clearer. Greater agreement and harmonization between clinical trialists, industry sponsors, and regulatory agencies will be required to evaluate new therapies in the most efficient way possible.

SUMMARY

The appropriate selection of response variables for AHF clinical trials is a complex process with major trade-offs. Reliance on short-term hemodynamic benefits or other surrogate end points has sidetracked AHF therapeutic development and treatment for decades, and as such is clearly unacceptable as a means of establishing therapeutic value. Moving forward, phase 3 clinical trials in AHF will need to focus on measures that clearly reflect clinical efficacy: mortality, hospitalization, and formal measures of health status, which may include durable relief of symptoms. Simultaneously, an improved process to provide more rapid and accurate evidence of longer-term safety must complement these efforts; this will require large clinical trials to bring the field of AHF firmly into the mainstream of evidence-based medicine. Unfortunately, recent failure of the two largest AHF trials conducted to date (PROTECT and ASCEND-HF, which included clinically oriented primary end points) may make the AHF community reluctant to commit to such large trials until better preliminary data are available. This approach, ironically, will require ongoing reliance on surrogate end points, which have contributed to the current conundrum of AHF therapeutic development.

REFERENCES

1. Roger VL, Go AS, Lloyd-Jones DM, et al. Heart disease and stroke statistics—2011 update: a report from the American Heart Association. Circulation 2011;123(4):e18–209.
2. Hunt SA, Abraham WT, Chin MH, et al. 2009 focused update incorporated into the ACC/AHA 2005 Guidelines for the Diagnosis and Management of Heart Failure in Adults: a report of the American College of Cardiology Foundation/American Heart Association Task Force on Practice Guidelines: developed in collaboration with the International Society for Heart and Lung Transplantation. Circulation 2009; 119(14):e391–479.
3. Lindenfeld J, Albert NM, Boehmer JP, et al. HFSA 2010 Comprehensive Heart Failure Practice Guideline. J Card Fail 2010;16(6):e1–194.
4. Dickstein K, Cohen-Solal A, Filippatos G, et al. ESC Guidelines for the diagnosis and treatment of acute and chronic heart failure 2008: the Task Force for the Diagnosis and Treatment of Acute and Chronic Heart Failure 2008 of the European Society of Cardiology. Developed in collaboration with the Heart Failure Association of the ESC (HFA) and endorsed by the European Society of Intensive Care Medicine (ESICM). Eur Heart J 2008;29(19):2388–442.
5. Nieminen MS, Bohm M, Cowie MR, et al. Executive summary of the guidelines on the diagnosis and treatment of acute heart failure: the Task Force on Acute Heart Failure of the European Society of Cardiology. Eur Heart J 2005;26(4):384–416.
6. Allen LA, O'Connor CM. Management of acute decompensated heart failure. CMAJ 2007;176(6): 797–805.
7. Allen LA, Hernandez AF, O'Connor CM, et al. End points for clinical trials in acute heart failure syndromes. J Am Coll Cardiol 2009;53(24):2248–58.
8. Zanolla L, Zardini P. Selection of endpoints for heart failure clinical trials. Eur J Heart Fail 2003;5(6):717–23.
9. Jessup M. Defining success in heart failure: the endpoint mess. Circulation 2010;121(18):1977–80.
10. Felker GM, Maisel AS. Development of therapeutics for heart failure: a global rank end point for clinical trials of acute heart failure. Circ Heart Fail 2010;3: 643–6.
11. Felker GM, O'Connor CM, Braunwald E. Loop diuretics in acute decompensated heart failure: necessary? Evil? A necessary evil? Circ Heart Fail 2009;2(1):56–62.
12. Massie BM, O'Connor CM, Metra M, et al. Rolofylline, an adenosine A1-receptor antagonist, in acute heart failure. N Engl J Med 2010;363(15):1419–28.
13. Gheorghiade M, Konstam MA, Burnett JC Jr, et al. Short-term clinical effects of tolvaptan, an oral vasopressin antagonist, in patients hospitalized for heart failure: the EVEREST Clinical Status Trials. JAMA 2007;297(12):1332–43.
14. Konstam MA, Gheorghiade M, Burnett JC Jr, et al. Effects of oral tolvaptan in patients hospitalized for worsening heart failure: the EVEREST Outcome Trial. JAMA 2007;297(12):1319–31.
15. Chaudhry SI, Mattera JA, Curtis JP, et al. Telemonitoring in patients with heart failure. N Engl J Med 2010;363(24):2301–9.
16. Bourge RC, Abraham WT, Adamson PB, et al. Randomized controlled trial of an implantable continuous hemodynamic monitor in patients with advanced heart failure: the COMPASS-HF study. J Am Coll Cardiol 2008;51(11):1073–9.
17. Costanzo MR, Guglin ME, Saltzberg MT, et al. Ultrafiltration versus intravenous diuretics for patients hospitalized for acute decompensated heart failure. J Am Coll Cardiol 2007;49(6):675–83.
18. Chaudhry SI, Wang Y, Concato J, et al. Patterns of weight change preceding hospitalization for heart failure. Circulation 2007;116(14):1549–54.
19. Felker GM, Pang PS, Adams KF, et al. Clinical trials of pharmacological therapies in acute heart failure syndromes: lessons learned and directions forward. Circ Heart Fail 2010;3(2):314–25.
20. Jencks SF, Williams MV, Coleman EA. Rehospitalizations among patients in the Medicare fee-for-service program. N Engl J Med 2009;360(14):1418–28.

21. Yusuf S, Negassa A. Choice of clinical outcomes in randomized trials of heart failure therapies: disease-specific or overall outcomes? Am Heart J 2002; 143(1):22–8.

22. Cuffe MS, Califf RM, Adams KF Jr, et al, Outcomes of a Prospective Trial of Intravenous Milrinone for Exacerbations of Chronic Heart Failure I. Short-term intravenous milrinone for acute exacerbation of chronic heart failure: a randomized controlled trial. JAMA 2002;287(12):1541–7.

23. Hernandez AF, O'Connor CM, Starling RC, et al. Rationale and design of the Acute Study of Clinical Effectiveness of Nesiritide in Decompensated Heart Failure Trial (ASCEND-HF). Am Heart J 2009;157(2): 271–7.

24. O'Connor CM, Starling RC, Hernandez AF, et al. Effect of nesiritide in patients with acute decompensated heart failure. N Engl J Med 2011;365:32–43.

25. Sackner-Bernstein JD, Kowalski M, Fox M, et al. Short-term risk of death after treatment with nesiritide for decompensated heart failure: a pooled analysis of randomized controlled trials. JAMA 2005; 293(15):1900–5.

26. Sackner-Bernstein JD, Skopicki HA, Aaronson KD. Risk of worsening renal function with nesiritide in patients with acutely decompensated heart failure. Circulation 2005;111(12):1487–91.

27. Teerlink JR. Overview of randomized clinical trials in acute heart failure syndromes. Am J Cardiol 2005; 96(6A):59G–67G.

28. Center for Drug Evaluation and Research, United States Food and Drug Administration. 21CFR Part 314-Applications for FDA Approval to Market a New Drug or an Antibiotic Drug. Available at: http://www.fda.gov/Drugs/GuidanceComplianceRegulatoryInformation/default.htm. Accessed January 30, 2011.

29. Stevenson LW, Hellkamp AS, Leier CV, et al. Changing preferences for survival after hospitalization with advanced heart failure. J Am Coll Cardiol 2008;52(21):1702–8.

30. Hohnloser SH, Kuck KH, Dorian P, et al. Prophylactic use of an implantable cardioverter-defibrillator after acute myocardial infarction. N Engl J Med 2004; 351(24):2481–8.

31. Fox CS, Evans JC, Larson MG, et al. A comparison of death certificate out-of-hospital coronary heart disease death with physician-adjudicated sudden cardiac death. Am J Cardiol 2005;95(7):856–9.

32. Mahaffey KW, Harrington RA, Akkerhuis M, et al. Systematic adjudication of myocardial infarction end-points in an international clinical trial. Curr Control Trials Cardiovasc Med 2001;2(4):180–6.

33. O'Connor CM, Miller AH, Konstam MA, et al. Mode of death and cardiovascular re-hospitalization in patients admitted with acute heart failure—results from the EVEREST program. Eur Heart J 2008; 7(Suppl):59–60.

34. Carson P, Anand I, O'Connor C, et al. Mode of death in advanced heart failure: the Comparison of Medical, Pacing, and Defibrillation Therapies in Heart Failure (COMPANION) trial. J Am Coll Cardiol 2005;46(12):2329–34.

35. Solomon SD, Anavekar N, Skali H, et al. Influence of ejection fraction on cardiovascular outcomes in a broad spectrum of heart failure patients. Circulation 2005;112(24):3738–44.

36. Zile MR, Gaasch WH, Anand IS, et al. Mode of death in patients with heart failure and a preserved ejection fraction: results from the Irbesartan in Heart Failure With Preserved Ejection Fraction Study (I-Preserve) trial. Circulation 2010;121(12):1393–405.

37. Lewis EF, Johnson PA, Johnson W, et al. Preferences for quality of life or survival expressed by patients with heart failure. J Heart Lung Transplant 2001; 20(9):1016–24.

38. Stewart GC, Brooks K, Pratibhu PP, et al. Thresholds of physical activity and life expectancy for patients considering destination ventricular assist devices. J Heart Lung Transplant 2009;28(9):863–9.

39. Spertus JA. Evolving applications for patient-centered health status measures. Circulation 2008; 118(20):2103–10.

40. The EQ-5D: an instrument designed to describe and value health. Available at: www.euroqol.org. Accessed December 18, 2010.

41. Utility assessment of health related quality of life. Available at: www.healthutilities.com. Accessed December 18, 2010.

42. The Short Form 36. Available at: www.sf-36.org. Accessed December 18, 2010.

43. Green CP, Porter CB, Bresnahan DR, et al. Development and evaluation of the Kansas City Cardiomyopathy Questionnaire: a new health status measure for heart failure. J Am Coll Cardiol 2000; 35(5):1245–55.

44. Spertus JA, Tooley J, Jones P, et al. Expanding the outcomes in clinical trials of heart failure: the quality of life and economic components of EPHESUS (EPlerenone's neuroHormonal Efficacy and SUrvival Study). Am Heart J 2002;143(4):636–42.

45. Rector TS, Kubo SH, Cohn JN. Validity of the Minnesota living with heart failure questionnaire as a measure of therapeutic response to enalapril or placebo. Am J Cardiol 1993;71(12):1106–7.

46. Spertus J, Peterson E, Conard MW, et al. Monitoring clinical changes in patients with heart failure: a comparison of methods. Am Heart J 2005;150(4): 707–15.

47. Soto GE, Jones P, Weintraub WS, et al. Prognostic value of health status in patients with heart failure after acute myocardial infarction. Circulation 2004; 110(5):546–51.

48. Kosiborod M, Soto GE, Jones PG, et al. Identifying heart failure patients at high risk for near-term

cardiovascular events with serial health status assessments. Circulation 2007;115(15):1975–81.

49. Heidenreich PA, Spertus JA, Jones PG, et al. Health status identifies heart failure outpatients at risk for hospitalization or death. J Am Coll Cardiol 2006; 47(4):752–6.

50. Chan PS, Soto G, Jones PG, et al. Patient health status and costs in heart failure: insights from the eplerenone post-acute myocardial infarction heart failure efficacy and survival study (EPHESUS). Circulation 2009;119(3):398–407.

51. Zuluaga MC, Guallar-Castillon P, Lopez-Garcia E, et al. Generic and disease-specific quality of life as a predictor of long-term mortality in heart failure. Eur J Heart Fail 2010;12(12):1372–8.

52. McMurray JJ, Teerlink JR, Cotter G, et al. Effects of te-zosentan on symptoms and clinical outcomes in patients with acute heart failure: the VERITAS random-ized controlled trials. JAMA 2007;298(17):2009–19.

53. Publication Committee for the VMAC Investigators (Vasodilatation in the Management of Acute CHF). Intravenous nesiritide vs nitroglycerin for treatment of decompensated congestive heart failure: a random-ized controlled trial. JAMA 2002;287(12):1531–40.

54. Pang PS, Cleland JG, Teerlink JR, et al. A proposal to standardize dyspnoea measurement in clinical trials of acute heart failure syndromes: the need for a uniform approach. Eur Heart J 2008;29(6):816–24.

55. Mahler DA, Weinberg DH, Wells CK, et al. The measurement of dyspnea. Contents, interobserver agreement, and physiologic correlates of two new clinical indexes. Chest 1984;85(6):751–8.

56. Mahler DA, Rosiello RA, Harver A, et al. Comparison of clinical dyspnea ratings and psychophysical measure-ments of respiratory sensation in obstructive airway disease. Am Rev Respir Dis 1987;135(6):1229–33.

57. Allen LA, Metra M, Milo-Cotter O, et al. Improvements in signs and symptoms during hospitalization for acute heart failure follow different patterns and depend on the measurement scales used: an interna-tional, prospective registry to evaluate the evolution of measures of disease severity in acute heart failure (MEASURE-AHF). J Card Fail 2008;14(9):777–84.

58. The Criteria Committee of the New York Heart Asso-ciation. Nomenclature and criteria for diagnosis of diseases of the heart and blood vessels. Boston: Little Brown; 1964.

59. Rafeal C, Briscoe C, Davies J, et al. Limitations of the New York Heart Association functional classifica-tion system and self-reported walking distances in chronic heart failure. Heart 2007;93(4):476–82.

60. Bennett JA, Riegel B, Bittner V, et al. Validity and reli-ability of the NYHA classes for measuring research outcomes in patients with cardiac disease. Heart Lung 2002;31(4):262–70.

61. Porter ME. What is value in health care? N Engl J Med 2010;363(26):2477–81.

62. Weinstein MC, Skinner JA. Comparative effective-ness and health care spending–implications for reform. N Engl J Med 2010;362(5):460–5.

63. Liao L, Allen LA, Whellan DJ. Economic burden of heart failure in the elderly. Pharmacoeconomics 2008;26(6):447–62.

64. Blair JE, Zannad F, Konstam MA, et al. Continental differences in clinical characteristics, management, and outcomes in patients hospitalized with wors-ening heart failure results from the EVEREST (Effi-cacy of Vasopressin Antagonism in Heart Failure: outcome study with Tolvaptan) program. J Am Coll Cardiol 2008;52(20):1640–8.

65. Nieminen MS, Brutsaert D, Dickstein K, et al. Euro-Heart Failure Survey II (EHFS II): a survey on hospi-talized acute heart failure patients: description of population. Eur Heart J 2006;27(22):2725–36.

66. Carson P, Fiuzat M, O'Connor C, et al. Determination of hospitalization type by investigator case report form or adjudication committee in a large heart failure clinical trial (beta-Blocker Evaluation of Survival Trial [BEST]). Am Heart J 2010;160(4): 649–54.

67. The Escape Investigators and Escape Study Coordi-nators. Evaluation study of congestive heart failure and pulmonary artery catheterization effectiveness: The ESCAPE Trial. JAMA 2005;294(13):1625–33.

68. Packer M. Randomized multicenter evaluation of intravenous levosimendan efficacy versus placebo in the short-term treatment of decompensated heart failure study (REVIVE-2). Paper presented at confer-ence: Proceedings of the American Heart Asso-ciation Scientific Sessions. Dallas (TX), November 13–16, 2005.

69. Committee for Medicinal Products for Human Use, European Medicines Agency. Note for guidance on clinical investigation of medicinal products for the treatment of cardiac failure: Addendum on Acute Cardiac Failure (CPMP/EWP/2986/03). 2004. Avail-able at: http://www.ema.europa.eu/docs/en_GB/document_library/Scientific_guideline/2009/09/WC500003338.pdf. Accessed July 11, 2011.

70. Ronco C, Haapio M, House AA, et al. Cardiorenal syndrome. J Am Coll Cardiol 2008;52(19):1527–39.

71. Fonarow GC, Adams KF Jr, Abraham WT, et al. Risk stratification for in-hospital mortality in acutely de-compensated heart failure: classification and regression tree analysis. JAMA 2005;293(5):572–80.

72. Prentice RL. Surrogate endpoints in clinical trials: definition and operational criteria. Stat Med 1989; 8(4):431–40.

73. Bucher HC, Guyatt GH, Cook DJ, et al. Users' guides to the medical literature: XIX. Applying clin-ical trial results. A. How to use an article measuring the effect of an intervention on surrogate end points. Evidence-Based Medicine Working Group. JAMA 1999;282(8):771–8.

74. Gerstein HC, Miller ME, Byington RP, et al. Effects of intensive glucose lowering in type 2 diabetes. N Engl J Med 2008;358(24):2545–59.

75. Kastelein JJ, Akdim F, Stroes ES, et al. Simvastatin with or without ezetimibe in familial hypercholesterolemia. N Engl J Med 2008;358(14):1431–43.

76. Braunwald E. Biomarkers in heart failure. N Engl J Med 2008;358(20):2148–59.

77. Xue Y, Clopton P, Peacock WF, et al. Serial changes in high-sensitive troponin I predict outcome in patients with decompensated heart failure. Eur J Heart Fail 2011;13(1):37–42.

78. Mebazaa A, Nieminen MS, Packer M, et al. Levosimendan vs dobutamine for patients with acute decompensated heart failure: the SURVIVE Randomized Trial. JAMA 2007;297(17):1883–91.

79. Cotter G, Dittrich HC, Weatherley BD, et al. The PROTECT pilot study: a randomized, placebo-controlled, dose-finding study of the adenosine A1 receptor antagonist rolofylline in patients with acute heart failure and renal impairment. J Card Fail 2008; 14(8):631–40.

80. U.S. Department of Health and Human Services, Food and Drug Administration. Guidance for industry: patient-reported outcome measures: use in medical product development to support labeling claims. December 2009. Available at: http://www.fda. gov/downloads/Drugs/GuidanceComplianceRegula toryInformation/Guidances/UCM193282.pdf. Accessed January 31, 2011.

81. Efficacy and safety of relaxin for the treatment of acute heart failure (RELAX-AHF). Available at: http://clinicaltrials.gov/ct2/show/NCT00520806. Accessed January 31, 2011.

82. Teerlink JR, Metra M, Felker GM, et al. Relaxin for the treatment of patients with acute heart failure (Pre-RELAX-AHF): a multicentre, randomised, placebo-controlled, parallel-group, dose-finding phase IIb study. Lancet 2009;373(9673): 1429–39.

Covariate Adjustment in Heart Failure Randomized Controlled Clinical Trials: A Case Analysis of the HF-ACTION Trial

Christopher M. O'Connor, MD[a],*, Robert J. Mentz, MD[b],
David J. Whellan, MD[c]

KEYWORDS

- Heart failure • Covariate adjustment • Clinical trials
- HF-ACTION

Randomized controlled clinical trials are the principal form of investigation to determine whether a therapeutic intervention is beneficial in patients with congestive heart failure (HF).[1,2] In the design and conduct of clinical trials, using large sample sizes is expected to protect against the imbalances among baseline characteristics that may influence outcome.[2] However, small differences that accumulate through multiple covariates can occur and, although not achieving statistical significance, may be important.[3] Therefore, clinical trialists have used several techniques, such as covariate analysis, to prevent imbalances from disturbing the overall results of randomized controlled clinical trials.[4] This article reviews the HF-ACTION trial to better understand whether covariate adjustment should be pre-specified as the primary end point in HF clinical trials.

ADJUSTMENT IN RANDOMIZED CONTROLLED TRIALS

Treatment effect adjustment has the goal of refining the analysis of an overall treatment difference through taking into account baseline characteristics that may be imbalanced between treatment groups.[3] These adjustments can be conducted and addressed in several different ways (**Box 1**).[4] Often an adjustment is made based on a stratification to prevent an imbalance in randomization in a single important covariate that is believed to be potentially important and perhaps has a differential effect size with therapeutic intervention[5] (**Fig. 1**). For example, in the PRAISE-I study evaluating amlodipine in the treatment of HF, patients were stratified based on whether the origin was ischemic or nonischemic, and a highly statistically significant effect on outcome was seen based on this difference.[6] Subsequently, trials of HF have commonly stratified patients based on etiology because of the differential effect on outcomes and event rates, and the uncoupling with therapy that has been seen in clinical trials.[7] The trialists have also stratified based on clinical site and sometimes regions of the world[8] to try to better prevent imbalances in recruitment sites or regions of the world where there may be asymmetric recruitment rates and differential clinical characteristics.

[a] Division of Cardiology, Duke University Medical Center, DUMC 3356, Durham, NC 27710, USA
[b] Department of Cardiology, Department of Medicine, Duke University Medical Center, 2301 Erwin Road, Durham, NC 27705, USA
[c] Division of Cardiology, Department of Medicine, Clinical Outcomes Research and Education, Jefferson Coordinating Center for Clinical Research, Jefferson Medical College, Thomas Jefferson University, 1015 Chestnut Street, Suite 317, Philadelphia, PA 19107, USA
* Corresponding author.
E-mail address: oconn002@mc.duke.edu

Heart Failure Clin 7 (2011) 497–500
doi:10.1016/j.hfc.2011.06.011
1551-7136/11/$ – see front matter © 2011 Published by Elsevier Inc.

A second more common adjustment method is based on a prespecified list of baseline covariates that may range from 2 to 10.[3,9,10] These variables often involve demographics, such as age, gender, and race, but also other important clinical characteristics known to effect prognosis in HF, such as New York Heart Association (NYHA) class, left ventricular ejection fraction, systolic blood pressure, and several biologic markers, such as blood urea nitrogen or creatinine, serum sodium, or hemoglobin, and brain natriuretic peptide if measured. These characteristics have been shown to be independently prognostically important and have been used for adjustment, usually in a secondary analysis.[1]

Finally, a third method of adjustment is based on prognostically important variables that may not have been fully identified at initiation of the protocol. In this form of covariate adjustment, after the database is locked but before the blind is broken, a full adjustment model is constructed to understand the important clinical predictors of the primary end point in the clinical trial's dataset (**Fig. 1**). In this situation, previously prespecified characteristics commonly enter as important predictors in the model in addition to previously unknown or unprespecified characteristics that emerge as statistically and clinically important from a prognostic standpoint.

The Importance of Adjustment

Covariate adjustment may provide more individualized effect estimates, especially in nonlinear models such as logistic regression and Cox proportional hazards regression, and the potential

exists for an improvement in power and a reduction in type I error.[4] Several studies have shown that covariate adjustment increases the power of statistical analysis of the treatment effect in the context of the randomized controlled trial without an increased risk in type I error.[4,11] This increase in power could allow for several important optimizations in a clinical trial, including (1) a reduced need for a large sample size, (2) an increase in the effect size, and (3) an increase in the level of statistical significance.

Because HF affects such a heterogeneous population, prespecifying an adjusted estimate for the primary analysis would seem to increase the precision of the clinical trial results. The observation that the effect of non–statistically significant imbalances between groups is not negligible, especially if their prognostic effect is strong,[3] further emphasizes the potential role for coadjusted analysis. Thus, the authors believe that one of the many lessons learned from the HF-ACTION trial is to prespecify, as the primary analysis, a covariate-adjusted analysis.

HF-ACTION

The HF-ACTION trial was a multicentered randomized controlled trial of 2331 medically stable patients with HF and reduced ejection fraction.[12] This trial was conducted from April 2003 through February 2007 at 82 centers within the United States, Canada, and France, and had a median follow-up of 30 months. The main outcome measure was a composite primary end point of all-cause mortality or hospitalization with prespecified secondary end points of all-cause mortality, cardiovascular mortality or hospitalization, and cardiovascular mortality or heart failure hospitalization. The study was designed to have a 90% power to detect an 11% reduction in the 2-year rate of all-cause mortality and hospitalization for patients randomized to exercise training compared with those randomized to usual care. The estimate was based on assuming the annual primary outcome rate of 30% of the usual group, treatment nonadherence rates of 30% during the first year of follow-up and 12.5% annually thereafter, and an annual crossover rate of 5% of the usual care group, with a planned median follow-up at 2.5 years and an alpha level of 0.05.[13]

Baseline patient characteristics were summarized using medians and interquartile ranges for continuous variables and frequencies and percentages for categorical variables, cumulative event rates were calculated using the Kaplan-Meier Method, and censoring times for all patients were measured from the time of randomization (time 0). All information available and the primary

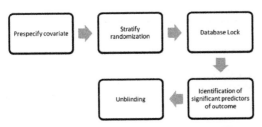

Fig. 1. Post-database lock, blinded covariate determination and adjustment.

Box 2
Examples of adjustment used in HF-ACTION

- Stratified enrollment
  - Ischemic vs nonischemic etiology of HF
- Prespecified baseline covariate adjustment
  - Age
  - Sex
  - Race
  - Previous myocardial infarction
  - Prior revascularization
  - NYHA functional class
  - Left ventricular ejection fraction
  - Ischemic vs nonischemic etiology
  - Baseline use of ß-blockers and angiotensin-converting enzyme inhibitors
- Postdatabase lock, blinded covariate determination, and adjustment
  - Duration at cardiopulmonary exercise test
  - Left ventricular ejection fraction
  - Beck Depression Inventory II score
  - History of atrial fibrillation or flutter

The Cox model was used to assess the consistency of the treatment effect through testing for interactions between treatment and prespecified baseline characteristics (**Box 2**).[13]

As specified in the HF-ACTION protocol, supplemental analysis of the primary end point and the secondary end points was performed adjusting for baseline characteristics predictive of the clinical outcomes. Time-to-event outcome adjustments for strong predictors of the outcomes enabled the analysis to more specifically compare patients with similar risks and thereby increase statistical power.[3] The baseline predictors of the primary outcome of all-cause mortality and hospitalization were objectively selected using stepwise variable selection based on treatment-blinded data. To avoid introducing bias to the variables selected, the authors were required to have little or no missing data, use only the most highly significant variables with all P values less than .001, and appropriately identify the process that was used in covariate-adjusted treatment comparisons.

Four baseline characteristics were identified as highly prognostic of the primary end point independent of treatment assignment (see **Box 2**): the duration at cardiopulmonary exercise test, left ventricular ejection fraction, Beck Depression Inventory score, and a history of atrial fibrillation or flutter. HF etiology as ischemic versus nonischemic was not identified as a significant predictor of the primary endpoint but was forced into the model as a covariate since it was the only factor selected for stratifying enrollment. After adjusting for these covariates the results were reported. **Table 1** shows the outcomes presented as unadjusted and adjusted for stratification effect. An important change is seen in all of the hazard ratios in the same direction, taking the P value

and secondary end points were connected to the final contact with the patient, including patients who withdrew consent or were lost to follow-up. The log-rank test was used to statistically compare the study groups with respect to the time to first occurrence of either component of the primary end point, and the secondary time-to-event outcomes, adjusting for HF etiology. Relative risks were expressed as hazard ratios and 95% CIs.

Table 1
Clinical events in HF-ACTION presented as unadjusted and adjusted for stratification effect

Event	% of Patients		Unadjusted HR (95% CI)	P Value for Unadjusted Analysis	Adjusted HR (95% CI)	P Value for Adjusted Analysis
	Usual Care (n = 1171)	Exercise Training (n = 1159)				
All-cause mortality or hospitalization (primary end point)	68	65	0.93 (0.84–1.02)	0.13	0.89 (0.81–0.99)	0.03[a]
CV mortality or hospitalization	58	55	0.92 (0.83–1.03)	0.14	0.91 (0.82–1.01)	0.09
CV mortality or HF hospitalization	34	30	0.87 (0.75–1.00)	0.06	0.85 (0.74–0.99)	0.03[a]

Abbreviations: CI, confidence interval; CV, cardiovascular; HF, heart failure; HR, hazard ratio.
[a] Statistical significance at the prespecified alpha level of 0.05.

from a slight association to significant by the pre-specified level for the primary end point and the secondary end point of cardiovascular mortality or HF hospitalization. Because the association was close to the nominal prespecified P value of significance in the unadjusted analysis, the association became significant after adjustment. This case represents a truly important example of covariate adjustment. The interpretation of this trial has been difficult because the corrected P-value drops from above the level of significance at .05 to below the level of significance.

SUMMARY

Randomized controlled trials are expensive and of long duration, particularly in the area of outpatient heart failure.[14] However, given the extensive morbidity and mortality associated with this condition and many novel new therapies emerging, more suitable well-designed clinical trials must be designed. Methods that can allow for greater precision and power and thus result in reduced sample sizes would be welcomed as a major event in clinical trial methodology.[14] In the HF-ACTION trial, the sample size was reduced from 3000 to 2331 because of a higher than expected event rate in all the participants. The trial results in the unadjusted and adjustment-for-strata-only analyses resulted in a nonsignificant statistical trend. Interpretation of this has led many people to believe that exercise has no role in HF management. However, given the foresight of the statistical and analytical team in the clinical trial, a prespecified covariate adjustment analysis was incorporated into the statistical and analytical clinical plan. This adjustment showed achievement of statistical significance for the primary and secondary end points of the trial, and thus has allowed the interpretation that exercise training did have a modest affect on improved clinical outcomes in HF. HF-ACTION is perhaps one of the best cases of a clinical trial in which covariate-adjusted analysis improved the precision of the trial. The HF-ACTION study stands as an important example of why covariate adjustment analysis should be considered as the primary method of analysis for the primary end point given the potential increase in statistical power.

REFERENCES

1. DeMets DL, Califf RM. Lessons learned from recent cardiovascular clinical trials: part II. Circulation 2002;106(7):880–6.

2. Yusuf S. Randomised controlled trials in cardiovascular medicine: past achievements, future challenges. BMJ 1999;319(7209):564–8.

3. Pocock SJ, Assmann SE, Enos LE, et al. Subgroup analysis, covariate adjustment and baseline comparisons in clinical trial reporting: current practice and problems. Stat Med 2002;21(19):2917–30.

4. Hernandez AV, Steyerberg EW, Habbema JD. Covariate adjustment in randomized controlled trials with dichotomous outcomes increases statistical power and reduces sample size requirements. J Clin Epidemiol 2004;57(5):454–60.

5. Kernan WN, Viscoli CM, Makuch RW, et al. Stratified randomization for clinical trials. J Clin Epidemiol 1999;52(1):19–26.

6. Packer M, O'Connor CM, Ghali JK, et al. Effect of amlodipine on morbidity and mortality in severe chronic heart failure. Prospective Randomized Amlodipine Survival Evaluation Study Group. N Engl J Med 1996;335(15):1107–14.

7. Felker GM, Benza RL, Chandler AB, et al. Heart failure etiology and response to milrinone in decompensated heart failure: results from the OPTIME-CHF study. J Am Coll Cardiol 2003;41(6):997–1003.

8. Weatherley BD, Cotter G, Dittrich HC, et al. Design and rationale of the PROTECT study: a placebo-controlled randomized study of the selective A1 adenosine receptor antagonist rolofylline for patients hospitalized with acute decompensated heart failure and volume overload to assess treatment effect on congestion and renal function. J Card Fail 2010;16(1):25–35.

9. Assmann SF, Pocock SJ, Enos LE, et al. Subgroup analysis and other (mis)uses of baseline data in clinical trials. Lancet 2000;355(9209):1064–9.

10. Senn S. Testing for baseline balance in clinical trials. Stat Med 1994;13(17):1715–26.

11. Roozenbeek B, Maas AI, Lingsma HF, et al. Baseline characteristics and statistical power in randomized controlled trials: selection, prognostic targeting, or covariate adjustment? Crit Care Med 2009;37(10):2683–90.

12. O'Connor CM, Whellan DJ, Lee KL, et al. Efficacy and safety of exercise training in patients with chronic heart failure: HF-ACTION randomized controlled trial. JAMA 2009;301(14):1439–50.

13. Whellan DJ, O'Connor CM, Lee KL, et al. Heart failure and a controlled trial investigating outcomes of exercise training (HF-ACTION): design and rationale. Am Heart J 2007;153(2):201–11.

14. Tunis SR, Stryer DB, Clancy CM. Practical clinical trials: increasing the value of clinical research for decision making in clinical and health policy. JAMA 2003;290(12):1624–32.

Biomarkers as Surrogate End Points in Heart Failure Trials

G. Michael Felker, MD, MHS

KEYWORDS

- Heart failure • Clinical trials • Surrogate end points
- Natriuretic peptides

Heart failure is among the most important public health problems in the developed world, with increasing prevalence, substantial morbidity and mortality, and high costs.[1] Despite improvements in therapy over recent decades, the overall prognosis of heart failure remains poor, with a projected median survival for symptomatic patients of less than 5 years. Although there have been important successes in the development of new therapies for chronic heart failure, recent trials have failed to show added benefit from new therapies.[2–6] In particular, there has been little progress in the development of new therapies for acute decompensated heart failure.[7] This lack of progress suggests the need for a critical reappraisal of the clinical research enterprise in heart failure, including clinical trial methodology. The topic of the most appropriate end points for heart failure studies is an ongoing subject of controversy and has recently been reviewed in detail.[8] Despite substantial interest in the development of surrogate end points for heart failure, none has been proven valid, a fact which has impaired the rapid evaluation of new heart failure therapies. This review focuses on the evidence supporting a potential role for biomarkers as surrogate end points in heart failure studies.

WHAT IS A BIOMARKER?

A biomarker has been defined as "a characteristic that is objectively measured and evaluated as an indicator of normal biological processes, pathogenic processes, or pharmacologic responses."[9] Although this definition is quite broad, for the purposes of this review the definition of biomarker is restricted to those markers that can be reproducibly measured in the blood or urine. Multiple biomarkers have been identified in heart failure and may reflect various underlying pathophysiologic processes.[10] Natriuretic peptides such as B-type natriuretic peptide (BNP) and its amino-terminal fragment the N-terminal pro B-type natriuretic peptide (NTproBNP) are well-established markers of ventricular wall stress.[11] Troponins play a central role in the diagnosis of acute coronary syndromes and are increasingly used in the management of patients with heart failure.[12] Novel markers, including ST-2,[13] galectin-3,[14] growth differentiation factor (GDF)-15,[15] mid-regional prohormone markers,[16] and others are emerging as potentially useful markers in heart failure. Although most of the research on biomarkers in heart failure has appropriately focused on their use as clinical tools, another emerging role of biomarkers is as part of the design and conduct of clinical trials. Based on their ability to assess underlying pathophysiologic processes in vivo in an objective, quantitative, and reproducible fashion, biomarkers have been viewed as potential surrogates for treatment effects. This article reviews the evidence for the validity of biomarkers, in particular the natriuretic peptides, as surrogates in heart failure clinical trials.

WHAT IS A SURROGATE?

A surrogate end point is defined as "a laboratory measurement or physical sign that is used in

Disclosures: Research funding and/or consulting from Roche Diagnostics, Amgen, Cytokinetics, BG Medicine, Otsuka, Corthera.
Duke Clinical Research Institute, 2400 Pratt Street, Room 0311 Terrace Level, Durham, NC 27705, USA
E-mail address: michael.felker@duke.edu

Heart Failure Clin 7 (2011) 501–507
doi:10.1016/j.hfc.2011.06.001

therapeutic trials as a substitute for a clinically meaningful end point that is a direct measure of how a patient feels, functions, or survives and is expected to predict the effect of the therapy".[9] Many physiologic variables have been suggested as possible surrogates in heart failure studies, including measures of functional capacity, ventricular function and volumes, hemodynamic changes, and biomarkers.

Determining whether a given end point is a surrogate or a clinical end point is not always straightforward. As an example, changes in a biomarker (eg, troponin) are now central to the diagnosis of acute myocardial infarction.[17] In the context of acute coronary syndrome studies, changes in a biomarker are considered clinical events and frequently represent most of the clinical events in a given study, often driving decisions about regulatory approval of new drugs.[18] In contrast, in heart failure trials changes in a biomarker (including troponin) are considered unproven surrogates and are not considered acceptable evidence of safety or efficacy.

Anand and colleagues[19] have defined 3 potential classes of surrogate end points in the context of drug development:

- *Strong surrogates:* a measure so clearly linked to the disease outcome of interest that changes in the surrogate are presumed to accurately and reliably reflect improvement in disease outcomes. Examples of this type of surrogate include the lowering of blood pressure for antihypertensive drugs. At present, no strong surrogates have been accepted for acute or chronic heart failure.
- *Developmental surrogates:* measures that are sufficiently linked to the disease outcome of interest that they can be used in the early phases (phase I and phase II studies) of drug development to look for signals of efficacy and/or establish preliminary evidence of the risk/benefit ratio.
- *Supportive surrogates:* measures that can provide supportive data to strengthen the biologic plausibility or perceived validity of other trial data. Supportive surrogates are often included as secondary end points in large clinical trials and provide supportive evidence for the primary analysis.

VALIDATING SURROGATES

Although the concept of surrogate end points is straightforward, validating surrogates for a given disease state remains a challenging problem. For a surrogate to be considered valid, several criteria must be met. A valid surrogate must have a consistent relationship with the outcome of interest across multiple studies. This step establishes an association but does not prove causality. Many variables that are considered to be predictors of prognosis in heart failure do not proceed past this step. As a second step toward establishing validity, changes in the putative surrogate end point should be associated with changes in the risk of developing the end point of interest. This relationship must be established across multiple studies and populations to be considered robust. There must be data supporting the concept that there is proportionality between changes in the surrogate and changes in the end point, ie, the magnitude of change in the surrogate is congruent with the magnitude of change in the end point.[19]

BIOMARKERS AS SURROGATES FOR EFFICACY: NATRIURETIC PEPTIDES

Of the available biomarkers in heart failure, the natriuretic peptides BNP and its amino-terminal fragment NT-proBNP have the most robust evidence linking them to outcomes and have been most often proposed as potential surrogates. As a case study of the challenges involved in evaluating surrogates, the evidence for the validity of natriuretic peptides as heart failure surrogates in the context of the previously outlined criteria is presented.

Natriuretic Peptides and Outcomes in Heart Failure

There is a robust body of evidence linking increases in natriuretic peptide levels to outcomes in heart failure. These have included studies in chronic heart failure,[20] acute decompensated heart failure,[21] heart failure with preserved ejection fraction,[22] and normal populations.[23] Few findings of association with outcome in cardiovascular disease are more robust than that of increased natriuretic peptide levels and adverse outcomes. In many datasets, baseline natriuretic peptide levels are the strongest overall predictor of risk of any available clinical or laboratory characteristic.[20,24] As described earlier, however, an association between a biomarker and outcome is insufficient to establish the validity of the biomarker as a surrogate end point.

Changes in Natriuretic Peptides and Outcomes in Heart Failure

An important aspect of evaluating the validity of a potential surrogate is establishing that changes in the surrogate are associated with changes in outcomes. Various observational studies have shown an association between decreasing natriuretic peptide levels over time and improved outcomes in both inpatients and outpatients with heart failure.[25–29] In a representative study of chronic heart failure, Masson and colleagues[29] examined the prognostic value of baseline and 4-month NT-proBNP values in a prospective substudy of patients enrolled in the placebo arm of the Valsartan Heart Failure Trial (Val-HeFT). This study demonstrated the powerful association of change in NT-proBNP levels over time with subsequent clinical outcomes. Using a cutoff point NT-proBNP level (derived from receiver operator analysis) of 1078 pg/mL, this study showed the prognostic significance of change in NT-proBNP values across this threshold over time. A similar analysis focused on BNP by Latini and colleagues[30] demonstrated substantially similar results based on changes more than and less than the median BNP level (97 pg/mL) (**Fig. 1**). Substantially similar data are available for shorter-term change in patients hospitalized with acute heart failure, demonstrating that patients whose natriuretic peptide level decreases during acute treatment have a much better prognosis than those whose natriuretic peptide level does not change.[25–27] These data provide broad evidence that changes in natriuretic peptide levels over time are one of the most powerful predictors of outcome in heart failure.

Changes in Natriuretic Peptides in Response to Proven Therapies

A large number of studies have also investigated the impact of proven heart failure therapies on natriuretic peptide levels. Therapies for heart failure proven to have beneficial long-term effects on morbidity and mortality, such as

angiotensin-converting enzyme inhibitors,[31] angiotensin receptor blockers,[32] beta-blockers,[33] aldosterone antagonists,[34] and cardiac resynchronization therapy,[35] all generally decrease natriuretic peptide levels. In Val-HeFT, the change in BNP was greater in patients randomized to valsartan (decrease by 34 pg/mL at 4 months) compared with those randomized to placebo (increase of 2 pg/mL at 4 months).[32] Similarly in the African-American Heart Failure Study, treatment with the combination of isosorbide dinitrate and hydralazine was associated with a larger reduction in BNP level at 6 months (39 pg/mL) compared with the placebo group (4 pg/mL).[36] Notably, in the Beta-blocker Evaluation of Survival Trial, bucindolol was not associated with improvement in BNP level compared with placebo,[37] which was consistent with the lack of efficacy of bucindolol on clinical outcomes.[38] Changes in natriuretic peptide levels in response to selected chronic therapies for heart failure are summarized in **Table 1**.

Can We Use Natriuretic Peptides as Surrogates for Efficacy in Heart Failure?

Based on the data outlined earlier, natriuretic peptides appear to fulfill many of the criteria for candidate surrogate end points in heart failure studies. However, the record on natriuretic peptide measurements as surrogate end points seems mixed. In the REVIVE trials of levosimendan in acute decompensated heart failure, treatment with levosimendan resulted in a significant decrease in BNP level compared with placebo for the 5 days after randomization. This short-term decrease in BNP level mirrored clinical improvement in the primary composite end point up to day 5.[39] However, despite these beneficial effects on natriuretic peptide levels and short-term outcomes, there was a trend towards increasing mortality in

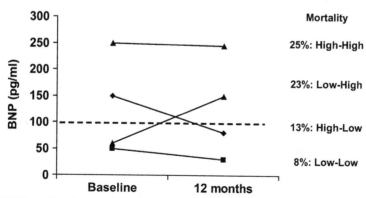

Fig. 1. Change in BNP from baseline to 12 months and relationship to mortality in patients enrolled in the VAL-HeFT study. (*From* Latini R, Masson S, Wong M, et al. Incremental prognostic value of changes in B-Type natriuretic peptide in heart failure. Am J Med 2006;119:70; with permission.)

Table 1
Changes in natriuretic peptides in selected clinical trials of chronic heart failure therapy

Trial	Treatment	Natriuretic Peptide	Time Interval (mo)	Treatment (pg/mL)	Placebo (pg/mL)
Val-HeFT[30]	Valsartan	BNP	3	−34	+2
A-HeFT[36]	Isosorbide and hydralazine	BNP	6	−39	−4
RALES[34]	Spironolactone	BNP	6	−15	−10
CARE-HF[35]	CRT	NT-proBNP	3	−808	−160
McMurray[42]	Aliskiren	NT-proBNP	3	−244	+762

Abbreviation: CRT, cardiac resynchronization therapy.

the levosimendan arm, which resulted in the drug not being approved in the United States. Similarly, in the SURVIVE trial comparing levosimendan with dobutamine, a short-term improvement in BNP levels with levosimendan therapy was not reflected in long-term survival benefits.[40] These data have led to continued uncertainty about the role of natriuretic peptide measurements as surrogate end points in heart failure.[41] One potentially useful distinction may be between surrogates for short-term treatment effect and surrogates for long-term safety. Short-term symptomatic improvement in acute heart failure is closely linked to hemodynamic improvements, which are typically reflected in natriuretic peptide levels. In contrast, long-term safety, which may be related to nonhemodynamic considerations (eg, myocardial injury, increased arrhythmias), would be unlikely to be captured by natriuretic peptide measurements.

Natriuretic peptide measurements continue to be explored as developmental surrogates to look for signals of efficacy earlier in the drug development process. An illustrative example is a study by McMurray and colleagues[42] examining the efficacy and safety of the direct renin inhibitor aliskiren versus placebo in 302 patients with chronic heart failure. This study evaluated changes in NT-proBNP plasma levels as the primary efficacy end point over 3 months. In this study, plasma NT-proBNP level increased by 762 pg/mL with placebo and decreased by 244 pg/mL with aliskiren ($P = 0.0106$). Similar findings were observed for BNP. Whether these changes in natriuretic peptides with therapy translate into clinical benefits is currently being tested in larger clinical trials, but these sort of data can provide early signals suggesting that development of a given drug candidate should proceed.

BIOMARKERS AS SURROGATES FOR SAFETY

Drug safety has become a major focus of drug development for both investigators and regulators.

The 2 most recent drugs approved for acute heart failure in the United States, milrinone and nesiritide, have both come under scrutiny because of concerns about adverse events and long-term safety.[43–45] The desire to identify safety concerns earlier in the process of drug development has led to the search for safety surrogates, measures that could reliably identify drugs with safety concerns. Because biomarkers reflect specific pathophysiologic processes, they may be well suited to play a role in identifying safety concerns in the drug development process. For example, increase in troponin levels has been shown to be a powerful predictor of adverse outcomes.[46,47] Preliminary data from small studies suggest that the development of new increase in troponin levels is a strong predictor of adverse events and heart failure progression in both acute[48] and chronic heart failure.[49] Newer ultrasensitive troponin assays will increase the potential to quantify the time course and extent of myocardial injury in patients with heart failure.[50] Although much about the mechanisms and timing of myocardial injury in acute heart failure remains uncertain, drugs that lead to myocardial injury seem unlikely to be safe and efficacious in the treatment of heart failure. Because safety in this context is really the absence of harm, so-called safety surrogates might be better characterized as harm surrogates. A drug that causes myocardial injury seems unlikely to have a favorable safety profile, but the absence of myocardial injury does not guarantee safety. This general concept has been piloted in early-phase heart failure studies, and the concept of drug-induced myocardial injury has recently been proposed as an important component of drug development in disease states other than ischemic heart disease.[51,52]

SUMMARY

Biomarkers play an increasingly important role in the management of patients with heart failure. In addition to their role as clinical tools, they are frequently incorporated into the design and conduct of clinical trials. Biomarkers such as natriuretic peptides have many attractive features as surrogate end points, particularly in early-phase studies. The potential use of natriuretic peptides (or any other biomarker) as surrogates in clinical trials must seek to align the pathophysiology of the surrogate with the pathophysiology of the end point for which it is a substitute. For example, biomarkers that reflect hemodynamic stress, such as natriuretic peptides, may serve as useful surrogates for clinical end points closely related to hemodynamic stress (eg, symptoms), but they are less valid for end points reflecting other processes (eg, sudden death). Ongoing development and validation of new markers that reflect disparate underlying mechanisms are likely to identify additional potential surrogates, and a multimarker approach to end points may be preferred to single biomarker surrogates. Despite the potential promise of biomarkers as surrogates, their validity remains unproven. Hence, the ultimate test of a therapy for a highly morbid condition such as heart failure remains its ability to improve either the quality or quantity of life; ie, it must make patients feel better and/or live longer.

REFERENCES

1. Lloyd-Jones D, Adams R, Carnethon M, et al. Heart disease and stroke statistics–2009 update: a report from the American Heart Association Statistics Committee and Stroke Statistics Subcommittee. Circulation 2009;119(3):e21–181.
2. McMurray JJ, Teerlink JR, Cotter G, et al. Effects of tezosentan on symptoms and clinical outcomes in patients with acute heart failure: the VERITAS randomized controlled trials. JAMA 2007;298(17):2009–19.
3. Mebazaa A, Nieminen MS, Packer M, et al. Levosimendan vs dobutamine for patients with acute decompensated heart failure: the SURVIVE Randomized Trial. JAMA 2007;297(17):1883–91.
4. Metra M, Eichhorn E, Abraham WT, et al. Effects of low-dose oral enoximone administration on mortality, morbidity, and exercise capacity in patients with advanced heart failure: the randomized, double-blind, placebo-controlled, parallel group ESSENTIAL trials. Eur Heart J 2009;30(24):3015–26.
5. Fox K, Ford I, Steg PG, et al. Ivabradine for patients with stable coronary artery disease and left-ventricular systolic dysfunction (BEAUTIFUL): a randomised, double-blind, placebo-controlled trial. Lancet 2008;372(9641):807–16.
6. Konstam MA, Gheorghiade M, Burnett JC Jr, et al. Effects of oral tolvaptan in patients hospitalized for worsening heart failure: the EVEREST Outcome Trial. JAMA 2007;297(12):1319–31.
7. Felker GM, Pang PS, Adams KF, et al. Clinical trials of pharmacological therapies in acute heart failure syndromes: lessons learned and directions forward. Circ Heart Fail 2010;3(2):314–25.
8. Allen LA, Hernandez AF, O'Connor CM, et al. End points for clinical trials in acute heart failure syndromes. J Am Coll Cardiol 2009;53(24):2248–58.
9. Atkinson AJ, Colburn WA, DeGruttola VG, et al. Biomarkers and surrogate endpoints: preferred definitions and conceptual framework. Clin Pharmacol Ther 2001;69(3):89–95.
10. Braunwald E. Biomarkers in heart failure. N Engl J Med 2008;358(20):2148–59.
11. Felker GM, Petersen JW, Mark DB. Natriuretic peptides in the diagnosis and management of heart failure. CMAJ 2006;175(6):611–7.
12. Miller WL, Hartman KA, Burritt MF, et al. Profiles of serial changes in cardiac troponin T concentrations and outcome in ambulatory patients with chronic heart failure. J Am Coll Cardiol 2009;54(18):1715–21.
13. Januzzi JL Jr, Peacock WF, Maisel AS, et al. Measurement of the interleukin family member ST2 in patients with acute dyspnea: results from the PRIDE (Pro-Brain Natriuretic Peptide Investigation of Dyspnea in the Emergency Department) study. J Am Coll Cardiol 2007;50(7):607–13.
14. van Kimmenade RR, Januzzi JL Jr, Ellinor PT, et al. Utility of amino-terminal pro-brain natriuretic peptide, galectin-3, and apelin for the evaluation of patients with acute heart failure. J Am Coll Cardiol 2006;48(6):1217–24.
15. Kempf T, von Haehling S, Peter T, et al. Prognostic utility of growth differentiation factor-15 in patients with chronic heart failure. J Am Coll Cardiol 2007;50(11):1054–60.
16. Maisel A, Mueller C, Nowak R, et al. Mid-region prohormone markers for diagnosis and prognosis in acute dyspnea: results from the BACH (Biomarkers in Acute Heart Failure) trial. J Am Coll Cardiol 2010;55(19):2062–76.
17. Thygesen K, Alpert JS, White HD, et al. Universal definition of myocardial infarction. Circulation 2007;116(22):2634–53.
18. Inhibition of platelet glycoprotein IIb/IIIa with eptifibatide in patients with acute coronary syndromes. The PURSUIT Trial Investigators. Platelet Glycoprotein IIb/IIIa in Unstable Angina: Receptor Suppression Using Integrilin Therapy. N Engl J Med 1998;339(7):436–43.
19. Anand IS, Florea VG, Fisher L. Surrogate end points in heart failure. J Am Coll Cardiol 2002;39(9):1414–21.
20. Cleland JG, McMurray JJ, Kjekshus J, et al. Plasma concentration of amino-terminal pro-brain natriuretic peptide in chronic heart failure: prediction of cardiovascular events and interaction with the effects of

rosuvastatin: a report from CORONA (Controlled Ro-suvastatin Multinational Trial in Heart Failure). J Am Coll Cardiol 2009;54(20):1850–9.

21. Januzzi JL Jr, Sakhuja R, O'Donoghue M, et al. Utility of amino-terminal pro-brain natriuretic peptide testing for prediction of 1-year mortality in patients with dyspnea treated in the Emergency Department. Arch Intern Med 2006;166(3):315–20.

22. Cleland JG, Taylor J, Tendera M. Prognosis in heart failure with a normal ejection fraction. N Engl J Med 2007;357(8):829–30.

23. Wang TJ, Larson MG, Levy D, et al. Plasma natriuretic peptide levels and the risk of cardiovascular events and death. N Engl J Med 2004;350(7):655–63.

24. Masson S, Latini R, Anand IS, et al. Direct compar-ison of B-type natriuretic peptide (BNP) and amino-terminal proBNP in a large population of patients with chronic and symptomatic heart failure: the Valsartan Heart Failure (Val-HeFT) data. Clin Chem 2006;52(8):1528–38.

25. Logeart D, Thabut G, Jourdain P, et al. Predischarge B-type natriuretic peptide assay for identifying patients at high risk of re-admission after decom-pensated heart failure. J Am Coll Cardiol 2004; 43(4):635–41.

26. Bettencourt P, Azevedo A, Pimenta J, et al. N-terminal-pro-brain natriuretic peptide predicts outcome after hospital discharge in heart failure patients. Circulation 2004;110(15):2168–74.

27. Metra M, Nodari S, Parrinello G, et al. The role of plasma biomarkers in acute heart failure. Serial changes and independent prognostic value of NT-proBNP and cardiac troponin-T. Eur J Heart Fail 2007;9(8):776–86.

28. Anand IS, Fisher LD, Chiang YT, et al. Changes in brain natriuretic peptide and norepinephrine over time and mortality and morbidity in the Valsartan Heart Failure Trial (Val-HeFT). Circulation 2003; 107(9):1278–83.

29. Masson S, Latini R, Anand IS, et al. Prognostic value of changes in N-terminal pro-brain natriuretic peptide in Val-HeFT (Valsartan Heart Failure Trial). J Am Coll Cardiol 2008;52(12):997–1003.

30. Latini R, Masson S, Wong M, et al. Incremental prog-nostic value of changes in B-type natriuretic peptide in heart failure. Am J Med 2006;119(1):70.

31. McKelvie RS, Yusuf S, Pericak D, et al. Comparison of candesartan, enalapril, and their combination in congestive heart failure: randomized evaluation of strategies for left ventricular dysfunction (RESOLVD) pilot study: the RESOLVD Pilot Study Investigators. Circulation 1999;100(10):1056–64.

32. Latini R, Masson S, Anand I, et al. Effects of valsar-tan on circulating brain natriuretic peptide and norepinephrine in symptomatic chronic heart failure: the Valsartan Heart Failure Trial (Val-HeFT). Circula-tion 2002;106(19):2454–8.

33. Frantz RP, Olson LJ, Grill D, et al. Carvedilol therapy is associated with a sustained decline in brain natri-uretic peptide levels in patients with congestive heart failure. Am Heart J 2005;149(3):541–7.

34. Rousseau MF, Gurné O, Duprez D, et al. Beneficial neurohormonal profile of spironolactone in severe congestive heart failure: results from the RALES neurohormonal substudy. J Am Coll Cardiol 2002; 40(9):1596–601.

35. Fruhwald FM, Fahrleitner-Pammer A, Berger R, et al. Early and sustained effects of cardiac resynchroni-zation therapy on N-terminal pro-B-type natriuretic peptide in patients with moderate to severe heart failure and cardiac dyssynchrony. Eur Heart J 2007;28(13):1592–7.

36. Cohn JN, Tam SW, Anand IS, et al. Isosorbide dini-trate and hydralazine in a fixed-dose combination produces further regression of left ventricular re-modeling in a well-treated black population with heart failure: results from A-HeFT. J Card Fail 2007; 13(5):331–9.

37. Frantz RP, Lowes BD, Grayburn PA, et al. Baseline and serial neurohormones in patients with conges-tive heart failure treated with and without bucindolol: results of the neurohumoral substudy of the Beta-Blocker Evaluation of Survival Study (BEST). J Card Fail 2007;13(6):437–44.

38. The Beta-Blocker Evaluation of Survival Trial Investi-gators. A trial of the beta-blocker bucindolol in patients with advanced heart failure. N Engl J Med 2001;344:1659–67.

39. Cleland JG, Freemantle N, Coletta AP, et al. Clinical trials update from the American Heart Association: REPAIR-AMI, ASTAMI, JELIS, MEGA, REVIVE-II, SURVIVE, and PROACTIVE. Eur J Heart Fail 2006; 8:105–10.

40. Cohen-Solal A, Logeart D, Huang B, et al. Lowered B-type natriuretic peptide in response to levosimen-dan or dobutamine treatment is associated with improved survival in patients with severe acutely de-compensated heart failure. J Am Coll Cardiol 2009; 53(25):2343–8.

41. Gheorghiade M, Pang PS. Are BNP changes during hospitalization for heart failure a reliable surrogate for predicting the effects of therapies on post-discharge mortality? J Am Coll Cardiol 2009; 53(25):2349–52.

42. McMurray JJV, Pitt B, Latini R, et al. Effects of the oral direct renin inhibitor aliskiren in patients with symp-tomatic heart failure. Circ Heart Fail 2008;1(1):17–24.

43. Cuffe MS, Califf RM, Adams KF Jr, et al. Short-term intravenous milrinone for acute exacerbation of chronic heart failure: a randomized controlled trial. JAMA 2002;287:1541–7.

44. Sackner-Bernstein JD, Kowalski M, Fox M, et al. Short-term risk of death after treatment with ne-siritide for decompensated heart failure: a pooled

analysis of randomized controlled trials. JAMA 2005; 293(15):1900–5.

45. Sackner-Bernstein JD, Skopicki HA, Aaronson KD. Risk of worsening renal function with nesiritide in patients with acutely decompensated heart failure. Circulation 2005;111(12):1487–91.

46. Horwich TB, Patel J, MacLellan WR, et al. Cardiac troponin I is associated with impaired hemodynamics, progressive left ventricular dysfunction, and increased mortality rates in advanced heart failure. Circulation 2003;108(7):833–8.

47. Peacock WF, De Marco T, Fonarow GC, et al. Cardiac troponin and outcome in acute heart failure. N Engl J Med 2008;358(20):2117–26.

48. Del Carlo CH, Pereira-Barretto AC, Cassaro-Strunz C, et al. Serial measure of cardiac troponin T levels for prediction of clinical events in decompensated heart failure. J Card Fail 2004;10(1):43–8.

49. Miller WL, Hartman KA, Burritt MF, et al. Serial biomarker measurements in ambulatory patients with chronic heart failure: the importance of change over time. Circulation 2007;116(3):249–57.

50. Latini R, Masson S, Anand IS, et al. Prognostic value of very low plasma concentrations of troponin T in patients with stable chronic heart failure. Circulation 2007;116(11):1242–9.

51. Berridge BR, Pettit S, Walker DB, et al. A translational approach to detecting drug-induced cardiac injury with cardiac troponins: consensus and recommendations from the Cardiac Troponins Biomarker Working Group of the Health and Environmental Sciences Institute. Am Heart J 2009;158(1):21–9.

52. Gheorghiade M, Gattis Stough W, Adams KF Jr, et al. The Pilot Randomized Study of Nesiritide Versus Dobutamine in Heart Failure (PRESERVD-HF). Am J Cardiol 2005;96(6A):18G–25G.

Imaging Surrogate End Points in Heart Failure Trials

Luca Bettari, MD[a],*, Salvador Borges-Neto, MD[b]

KEYWORDS

- Heart failure • Imaging biomarkers • Surrogate end points
- Clinical trials

Heart failure (HF) is a major and growing public health problem because of its prevalence, incidence, morbidity, mortality, and economic costs.[1] The mortality rate for HF remains more than 60% within 5 years of diagnosis,[2] and 50% of hospitalized HF patients require readmission within 6 months of discharge.[3] Despite the initial successes, recent trials have failed to show benefit from new therapies,[4] and have suggested the need for a critical reappraisal of clinical research and trial methodology in HF.[5] End-point selection is one of the most important topics of this discussion.[6] In this setting, biomarkers could be used as surrogate end points and substitute true end points, reducing the costs of the trials (eg, time and sample size reduction); however, none have been proved valid as yet (**Box 1**). This article explores the adequacy and potential role of several imaging biomarkers, in particular left ventricular (LV) dimensions and left ventricular ejection fraction (LVEF), to serve as surrogate end points for clinical outcome in acute HF trials.

WHAT IS A TRUE END POINT?

Because HF is a life-threatening and debilitating disorder, true end points in HF trials reflect duration and quality of life.

Survival

Mortality is the most important end point for evaluation and regulatory approval of new HF drugs and, although mortality is a strong and easily measured end point, it has several limitations. The main concern of using only all-cause and cardiovascular mortality as an end point is that it refers to the extreme manifestation of HF. Thus, some of the patients (those less sick) in the study might not contribute to the outcomes and yet might have important quality of life (QoL) issues. Moreover, trials using mortality as the primary end point require a large sample size to show a survival advantage.

Quality of Life

QoL questionnaires may provide comprehensive information about the effects of a disease and its treatment on patients' lives. However, few questionnaires have been validated in HF patients in a way that shows that the results correlate with the severity of disease.[7] Statistically significant improvements in the QoL score have been observed in several studies,[8] and some of these studies also demonstrated an adverse effect on survival,[9] raising the issue of a mismatch between improvements in QoL and increase in survival.

Disclosures: Dr Bettari has no relationship to disclose. Dr Borges-Neto is a consultant for GE Healthcare and Gilead, and received a grant from GE Healthcare (gs1) and Astellas Inc.
[a] Duke Clinical Research Institute, 2400 Pratt Street, Durham, NC 27705, USA
[b] Division of Cardiology, Duke University Medical Center, 2301 Erwin Road, Durham, NC 27710, USA
* Corresponding author.
E-mail address: luca_bettari@yahoo.it

Box 1
Definition of biomarkers, surrogate end points, and clinical end points

Biomarker

A characteristic that is objectively measured and evaluated as an indicator of normal biological processes, pathogenic processes, or pharmacologic responses to a therapeutic intervention

Surrogate end point

A biomarker intended to substitute for a clinical end point. It should predict clinical changes on the basis of epidemiologic, therapeutic, pathophysiological, or other scientific evidence

Changes in the biomarker that results from therapy are expected to reflect changes in clinically meaningful end points

Clinical end point

A characteristic or variable that reflects how a patient feels, functions, or survives

---

Increased mortality with these and other tools indicates that symptomatic benefit in HF does not necessarily predict improved survival.[10]

WHAT IS A BIOMARKER?

A biomarker has been defined as a characteristic that is objectively measured and evaluated as an indicator of normal biological processes, pathogenic processes, or pharmacologic responses.[11] The integration of biomarkers into drug trials may increase the efficiency of the drug development process by early identification of potential responders or patient subgroups at risk for specific side effects, counteracting the rising costs of drug development. For the purposes of this review the authors restrict the definition of biomarker to imaging biomarkers, which are defined as any anatomic, physiologic, biochemical, or molecular parameter detectable by one or more imaging methods used to establish the presence and/or severity of a disease.[12] Multiple imaging biomarkers have been identified in HF and may reflect a variety of underlying pathophysiologic processes[13]; for example, LV dimensions and LVEF are well-established markers used to assess function and prognosis of HF patients. Moreover, based on their ability to assess underlying pathophysiologic processes in objective, quantitative, and reproducible fashion, imaging biomarkers have been viewed as clinical tools and/or potential surrogate end points to evaluate the treatment effects in HF trials. For imaging biomarkers to be accepted as surrogate end points, considerable evidence is needed from clinical trials to assess and validate the relationship with the true clinical end point, and several criteria must be fulfilled: relevance, sensitivity, specificity for treatment effects, reliability, practicality, and efficiency.[14]

WHAT IS A SURROGATE END POINT?

A surrogate end point of a clinical trial is a laboratory measurement or a physical sign used as a substitute for a clinically meaningful end point that measures directly how a patient feels, functions, or survives.[11] Changes induced by therapy on a surrogate end point are expected to reflect changes in a clinically meaningful end point. Surrogate end points have several potential advantages: clinical trials evaluating surrogate end points require smaller sample size and may be completed in less time to prove or disprove a hypothesis. The ability to bring effective therapies to clinical practice in an appropriate timeframe as well as less expensively makes surrogate end points attractive in the drug-approval process. The principal disadvantage of using surrogates to assess therapies is the possibility of a misleading evaluation.[15] Many physiologic variables have been suggested as possible surrogate end points for HF trials, including measures of functional capacity, ventricular function, volumes, hemodynamic changes, and biomarkers.

Three potential classes of surrogate end points in the context of drug development have been identified[16]:

Strong surrogates: measurements clearly linked to the disease of interest that changes in the surrogate are presumed to accurately reflect changes in the true end point. At present, there are no strong surrogates with widespread acceptance for acute or chronic HF trials.

Developmental surrogates: measurements closely related to the disease of interest that can be used in early phases (phase 1 and 2 studies) of drug development for dose ranging, preliminary proof of efficacy, and risk/benefit ratio.

Supportive surrogates: measurements that strengthen the plausibility of favorable results from other controlled data. These types of surrogates are often included as secondary end points in large clinical trials and provide supportive evidence for the primary analysis.

HOW TO VALIDATE SURROGATE END POINTS

Although the concept of surrogate end points is straightforward, validating biomarkers as surrogate end points for a given disease remains a challenging problem. In order for a surrogate end point to be considered valid, several criteria must be met.[17] First, a surrogate end point must have a consistent relationship with the clinical outcome/end point of interest. This step establishes an association but does not prove causality. Many variables that are considered to be predictors of prognosis in HF do not proceed past this step. Second, changes in the surrogate end point should be associated with changes in the risk of developing the end point of interest independent of treatment. Third, a consistent proportionality between the degree of change in the surrogate end point and the true end point must be demonstrated, so that the magnitude of change in the surrogate end point can predict the change in the true end point (eg, change in LV volume and survival).[16] Finally, these associations need to be replicated in several different populations, in both observational studies and treatment trials, using different therapeutic interventions.

A more feasible expectation is that the surrogate end point accounts for a substantial portion of the treatment effect on the true clinical end point. A measurement can be proposed as surrogate end point when the variable meets two criteria[15]: first, a statistical relationship must exist between the change in the proposed surrogate end point over time and the clinical outcome; second, a pathophysiologic basis must exist for believing that the change in the surrogate end point is the primary determinant of the outcome. Thus, surrogate end points in HF patients should unequivocally reflect the true end points (ie, survival and QoL).

WHICH IMAGING BIOMARKERS COULD BE SURROGATE END POINTS?
Hemodynamic Parameters

Intracardiac pressure measurements, stroke volume and cardiac output, right atrial pressure, and pulmonary artery pressures all can be estimated noninvasively through echocardiography[18]; moreover, echocardiography can determine abnormal diastolic function, increased left atrial pressure, and LV end-diastolic pressure, and all of these measurements have demonstrated considerable prognostic value in HF patients.[19] The adverse prognosis associated with systolic dysfunction is well described, but isolated diastolic HF also carries a poor prognosis.[20] Persistence of a restrictive filling pattern (severe diastolic dysfunction) during the Valsalva maneuver or on follow-up echocardiogram after HF therapy portends a poor prognosis.[21] Additional parameters such as an abnormal ratio of the systolic (S) and diastolic (D) velocities of pulmonary venous inflow (S/D<1); a systolic fraction of pulmonary venous forward flow (SF) of less than 40%; and an early LV filling flow propagation slope (Vp) of less than 45 cm/s have also been shown to be reliable predictors of high LV filling pressures and cardiovascular mortality.[22] Of note, increased left atrial volumes (>32 mL/m^2) have been shown to predict morbidity.[23] Also of interest, the ratio of peak early mitral inflow velocity to peak early diastolic myocardial velocity (E/E') has proved superior to brain natriuretic peptide levels in diagnosing volume overload.[24]

Left Ventricular Dimensions and LVEF

Baseline LV dimensions and LVEF have been shown to be one of the most powerful predictors of survival in HF patients.[25] Many of the beneficial effects of angiotensin-converting enzyme inhibitors and β-blockers in HF appear to be related to the ability of these agents to inhibit or to reverse cardiac remodeling.[26] In the Survival And Ventricular Enlargement (SAVE) trial,[27] treatment with captopril was associated with attenuation of LV enlargement over time, and improved clinical outcome. Serial assessments of LV dimensions and function in the Studies of Left Ventricular Dysfunction (SOLVD), Australia-New Zealand Carvedilol Heart Failure and Carvedilol Post-Infarct Survival Control in Left Ventricular Dysfunction (CAPRICORN) echocardiographic substudies,[28,29] and the Metoprolol CR/XL Randomized Intervention Trial in Heart Failure (MERIT-HF) magnetic resonance imaging (MRI) substudy have also found an association between favorable changes in LV dimensions and LVEF and improved clinical outcome produced by enalapril, carvedilol, or metoprolol.[30,31] The prognostic value of serial changes in LVEF in HF patients has been evaluated in the Vasodilator Heart Failure Trials I and II (V-HeFT I-II), in which a significant and proportionate relationship between the direction and magnitude of changes in LVEF over time and the 1-year mortality was demonstrated. Changes in LVEF greater than 5% from baseline at 6 months (V-HeFT I) and 12 months (V-HeFT II) were the strongest predictors of mortality, and remained significant even after adjustment for therapy and baseline LVEF.[32] Thus, LV dimensions and LVEF seem to fulfill most of the criteria for surrogate end points: baseline LV dimensions and LVEF are significantly related to prognosis, changes in these measurements reflect changes in mortality, and both the direction and the magnitude of change in these variables cause a proportional change in survival.

However, there are also HF trials in which the change in LVEF determined by therapy has not been consistently correlated with clinical outcomes. For example, in trials of chronically administered inotropic agents (such as milrinone), it was shown that inotropic agents improved hemodynamic profiles, increasing cardiac output and, in some cases, LVEF.[33] However, in larger, long-term studies, these agents were associated with an adverse effect on mortality rates. Conversely, β-blockers, which initially decrease LVEF, have consistently been shown to improve LVEF, stimulate reverse remodeling, and improve survival rates over the long term. These observations lead to the conclusion that LVEF per se is neither a suitable surrogate end point nor a feasible replacement for the assessment of clinical outcomes. However, in phase 2 trials, change in LVEF is an attractive end point to measure because it is useful to understand the mechanism of action of new pharmacologic therapies.

In contrast to evaluating only measures of LVEF, measures of cardiac remodeling are gaining more interest. Agents that favorably affect remodeling or promote reverse remodeling also appear to have beneficial effects on clinical outcome. Although remodeling may be the most likely variable to consider as a reliable surrogate end point, a dissociation between LV remodeling and mortality was observed in the Randomized Evaluation of Strategies for Left Ventricular Dysfunction (RESOLVD) trial.[34] Of note, LV dyssynchrony was also evaluated by echocardiography to predict response to cardiac resynchronization therapy, but did not result in being predictive; moreover, there was disagreement between echocardiographic readers to adjudicate the presence of dyssynchrony. Definitive conclusions regarding LV remodeling as a surrogate end point cannot be made from this trial. Thus, LV remodeling has not been proved to serve as a legitimate surrogate end point and currently cannot replace scientifically valid assessments of clinical outcomes.

Tei Index

The myocardial performance index (Tei index) is a Doppler parameter that provides global assessment of systolic and diastolic function. The Tei index consists of the ratio of the isovolumic contraction + isovolumic relaxation times/ejection time. The Tei index is independent of heart rate and blood pressure, applies to left and right

ventricular systolic and diastolic dysfunction, does not rely on geometric assumptions, and is highly reproducible.[35] The prognostic value of the Tei index has been validated in patients with dilated cardiomyopathy (DCM), proving to be superior to LVEF in predicting cardiac death and disease severity.[36] Moreover, the Tei index has been proved as effective in predicting the lack of clinical response to treatment in a study including patients with systolic HF and HF with preserved LVEF.[37] Because adequate Doppler images can be acquired even when the image quality is suboptimal, the Tei index might be particularly useful when other measures of left and right ventricular function are indeterminate.

Left Ventricular Mass

Although LV mass has received less attention than LVEF, it is an important prognostic marker in HF patients with and without coronary artery disease (CAD).[38] This observation in smaller studies was confirmed in the echocardiographic substudy of the SOLVD registry and trials in which investigators examined the effect of LV hypertrophy on clinical outcomes, and found that increased LV mass was associated with high mortality and rate of cardiovascular hospital stays, independent of LVEF.[39] LV mass increases in the remodeled, failing heart, either from increased volumes with myocardial thinning or from wall hypertrophy in patients with hypertensive cardiomyopathy.[40] Thus, the assessment of LV mass seems to provide not only an important research tool to evaluate remodeling but also a precise and prognostically powerful way to characterize clinical status.

Left atrial (LA) size is considered a marker of poor prognosis in HF patients. The MeRGE collaboration combined prospective data from 18 studies in HF patients. This analysis of data from 1157 patients showed that at the multivariate analysis, LA area was associated with prognosis (hazard ratio 1.03 per cm^2, 95% confidence interval [CI] 1.02–1.05; $P<.0001$) independently of age, NYHA class, LVEF, and restrictive filling pattern (RFP). When LA area was used as a categorical variable, the hazard ratio associated with larger LA area (above median) was 1.4 (95% CI 1.13–1.74) and when LA area index was used, the hazard ratio was 2.36 (95% CI 1.80–3.08). When the patients with and without RFP were divided on the basis of either LA area or LA area index, significantly higher event rates were observed in those with larger LA area. Thus LA area is a powerful predictor of outcome among HF patients with predominantly impaired systolic function, and is independent of, and provides additional prognostic information beyond, LV systolic and diastolic function.[41]

Right Ventricular Ejection Fraction

Quantification of right ventricular (RV) ejection fraction by MRI late after acute myocardial infarction (AMI) has been demonstrated to be an important predictor of prognosis even after being adjusted for patient age, LV infarct size, and LVEF.[42]

Myocardial Motion, Strain, and Strain Rate

Tissue Doppler imaging, in particular the peak systolic myocardial velocity, which reflects longitudinal myocardial fiber shortening, has been used to assess systolic function in HF patients.[43] Systolic myocardial velocity might provide a more accurate measure of systolic dysfunction than LVEF[44]; moreover, in HF patients tissue velocity measures have demonstrated reliable prognostic ability compared with standard echocardiographic measures, including LVEF.[45] Tissue velocity measurements are susceptible to artifact from tethering and translational motion, but strain imaging, derived from tissue velocity measurements, overcomes this limitation by measuring actual deformation of the myocardium in systole and diastole.

Infarct Size

The dimension of the infarct scar determined by late gadolinium enhancement-magnetic resonance imaging (LGE-MRI) has been demonstrated to be a reliable predictor of inducible ventricular tachycardia in electrophysiological studies to an even greater extent than LVEF.[46] Moreover, the extent of the peri-infarct zone assessed by MRI has been related to all-cause mortality.[47] Of note, increased infarct tissue heterogeneity identified by MRI has been demonstrated to increase the susceptibility to ventricular arrhythmias in patients with prior AMI and LV dysfunction.[48]

Furthermore, single-photon emission computed tomography (SPECT) myocardial perfusion imaging defects have been shown to identify patients at high risk of cardiovascular events and cardiovascular mortality,[49] including those resuscitated from SCD,[50] and patients with CAD at risk for de novo SCD.[51]

Mehta and colleagues[52] evaluated the prognostic impact of RV myocardial involvement in patients with inferior AMI. The investigators examined the incidence of death and mechanical and electrical complications in patients with (491) and without (638) RV myocardial involvement and in patients with anterior AMI (971) in an analysis from the Collaborative Organization for RheothRx Evaluation (CORE) trial. LV infarct size was assessed by technetium-99m–sestamibi SPECT and peak creatine kinase, and LV function was assessed by radionuclide angiography. Mehta and colleagues also performed a meta-analysis in which they pooled the results of this study with previous smaller studies addressing the same question. Six-month mortality was 7.8% in inferior AMI compared with 13.2% in anterior AMI. Among patients with inferior AMI, serious arrhythmias were significantly more common in patients with RV myocardial involvement who also had a trend toward higher mortality, pump failure, and mechanical complications. However, this was not associated with a difference in LV infarct size or function. A meta-analysis of 6 studies (1198) confirmed that RV myocardial involvement was associated with an increased risk of death (odds ratio [OR] 3.2, 95% CI 2.4–4.1), shock (OR 3.2, 95% CI 2.4–3.5), ventricular tachycardia or fibrillation (OR 2.7, 95% CI 2.1–3.5), and atrioventricular block (OR 3.4, 95% CI 2.7–4.2). Thus the investigators concluded that patients with inferior myocardial infarction who also have RV myocardial involvement are at increased risk of death, shock, and arrhythmias ($P<.00001$ for all). This increased risk is related to the presence of RV myocardial involvement itself rather than the extent of LV myocardial damage.

Microvascular Dysfunction

It has been shown that in the absence of macroscopic CAD, global flow reserve can be impaired in HF patients as a consequence of microvascular dysfunction.[53] The concept of microvascular dysfunction (determined by positron emission tomography [PET]) as an independent contributor to the progression of HF in cardiomyopathy has been supported by several outcome studies.[54] Neglia and colleagues[54] demonstrated in 67 patients with idiopathic DCM that myocardial blood flow impairment (<1.36 mL/min/g) determined by rest-stress PET imaging protocol with $^{13}NH_3$ was predictive for adverse cardiac events.

Microvascular Obstruction

The obstruction of microcoronary circulation detected by MRI predicts aggravated ventricular remodeling and adverse cardiovascular events after AMI.[55] Among patients with a clinical suspicion of CAD but without a history of AMI, the identification of LGE involving even a small amount of myocardium carries a high risk of future cardiac events with incremental prognostic value beyond common clinical, angiographic, and functional predictors.[56]

Fibrosis

A pattern of this type in DCM patients with symptomatic HF was associated with a high rate of all-cause mortality and hospitalization even after adjustment for age, LV function, and ventricular volumes measured by MRI.[57] Furthermore, adverse cardiac prognosis in DCM patients is associated with the presence of LGE regardless of segmental pattern.[58] Patients who had LGE of any pattern showed an eightfold higher risk of reaching a composite outcome of HF hospitalization, appropriate implantable defibrillator discharges, and cardiac death compared with patients without LGE. Similar to findings in ischemic cardiomyopathy, the presence of scarring on LGE-MRI in DCM patients is predictive of inducible ventricular tachycardia even after adjustment for LVEF.[59]

Recently the results of the nuclear substudy of the HF-ACTION trial have been presented.[60] This substudy included 240 patients with LV dysfunction. Sum rest scores were obtained from 238 of these patients using gated SPECT. The primary end point was a combination of all-cause mortality and CV hospitalization. According to a Cox proportional hazards model based on 113 events occurring in 238 patients, the extent and severity of baseline perfusion abnormalities was a predictor of the combined end point (hazard ratio 0.98; 95% CI 0.97–1.00). However, the investigators also reported that a higher baseline sum rest score was associated with a lower risk for an event. The investigators explained the relationship by noting that the outcomes were driven by a small group of patients with ischemic cardiomyopathy. Patients with high sum rest scores at baseline who had ischemia were more likely to experience the primary end point than those without ischemic cardiomyopathy who had similar sum rest scores ($P = .008$ for interaction). This finding leads to the hypothesis that there is an inverse relationship between the degree and severity of resting perfusion abnormalities and mortality and CV hospitalization, and furthermore is related to ischemic events leading to CV hospitalization (which were the driven outcomes in the study) in patients with less severe resting perfusion abnormalities.

Sympathetic Innervation

HF patients with deprived cardiac sympathetic innervation tend to have a worse prognosis when compared with those with relatively preserved neuronal integrity.[61] Decreased myocardial iodine-123–metaiodobenzylguanidine ([123I]MIBG) uptake in HF patients has been consistently shown to be associated with poorer prognosis.[62] There is an increasing body of literature documenting an association between abnormalities of myocardial [123I]MIBG uptake and risk of ventricular arrhythmia and sudden cardiac death in patients with both ischemic and nonischemic cardiomyopathies.[63]

Moreover, studies have also shown that the rate in which [123I]MIBG is washout from the myocardium is important for prognosis stratification of HF patients.[64] Recently, the AdreView Myocardial Imaging for Risk Evaluation in Heart Failure (ADMIRE-HF) trial evaluated the prognostic value of cardiac [123I]MIBG planar computed tomography and SPECT imaging with imaging in 961 HF patients.[65] Patients with adverse events showed significantly lower early and late heart-to-mediastinum (H/M) ratio ($P<.01$) as well as higher myocardial washout rate ($P<.01$) than patients without adverse events during follow-up. Moreover, the risk for major cardiac events was significantly lower in patients with an H/M ratio of 1.60 or greater when compared with patients with an H/M ratio less than 1.60 (hazard ratio 0.40, 95% CI 0.25–0.64, $P<.01$).

Myocardial Viability

Several observational studies have suggested survival benefit in patients with severe CAD and LV dysfunction if they are revascularized when myocardial viability is detected on imaging tests. A meta-analysis by Allman and colleagues[66] pooled data from 24 viability studies reporting patient survival, using thallium perfusion imaging, fluorine-18 fluorodeoxyglucose metabolic imaging, or dobutamine echocardiography to examine late survival with revascularization versus medical therapy after myocardial viability testing. There were 3088 patients (mean LVEF 32% ± 8%) followed for 25 ± 10 months. In patients with viability, revascularization was associated with 79.6% reduction in annual mortality (16% vs 3.2%, $\chi^2 = 147$, $P<.0001$) compared with medical treatment. Patients without viability had intermediate mortality, trending to higher rates with revascularization versus medical therapy (7.7% vs 6.2%, $P =$ not significant). Patients with viability showed a direct relationship between severity of LV dysfunction and magnitude of benefit with revascularization ($P<.001$). There was no measurable performance difference for predicting revascularization benefit between the 3 testing techniques. This meta-analysis demonstrates a strong association between myocardial viability on noninvasive testing and improved survival after revascularization in patients with chronic CAD and LV dysfunction.

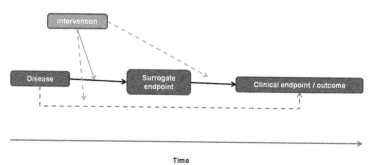

Time

Fig. 1. Possible relationships between disease, surrogate end point, and clinical end point.

Absence of viability was associated with no significant difference in outcomes, irrespective of treatment strategy.

POSSIBLE USE OF IMAGING SURROGATE END POINTS IN HF TRIALS

Imaging biomarkers serve different purposes in drug development.

In early clinical trials, imaging biomarkers can enhance product knowledge to elucidate the drug's potential in different patient groups and disease states. The information obtained at this stage is important for the design of subsequent clinical trials (ie, to identify promising drug candidates and to stop unpromising projects early).

In later clinical trials, imaging biomarkers have the potential to serve as surrogate end points and support approval for market use. Considerations regarding the selection of the best imaging biomarkers in the context of a trial include practical aspects such as the broad availability of the test method and the simplicity of its application. Therefore, technically or logistically demanding imaging techniques are less likely to serve as effective biomarkers in later clinical development. The value of imaging biomarkers as surrogate end points will be greatest in targeting specific compounds that are effective in a subgroup of patients only. Thus, appropriate use of biomarkers will help to identify in a clinical phase 2 trial those patient subgroups most likely to respond or to exhibit safety problems, and so streamline the clinical phase 3 trial.

SUMMARY

Imaging biomarkers play an increasingly important role in the management of HF patients. In addition to their role as clinical tools, they are frequently incorporated into the design and conduct of clinical trials. Imaging biomarkers such as LV dimensions and LVEF have many attractive features as surrogate end points, in particular for early-phase studies. The potential use of imaging biomarkers as surrogate end points in clinical trials must seek to align the pathophysiology of the surrogate with the pathophysiology of the clinical end point for which it is designed to substitute (**Fig. 1**). For example, imaging biomarkers that reflect hemodynamic improvement (eg, LVEF) may serve as a useful surrogate for clinical end points closely related to hemodynamic improvement (eg, symptoms), but are less valid for clinical end points reflecting other processes (eg, long-tem mortality). Ongoing development and validation of new biomarkers that reflect disparate underlying mechanisms is likely to identify additional potential surrogate end points, and a "multimarker" approach to end points may be preferred to single-biomarker surrogate end points. Despite the potential promise of imaging biomarkers as surrogate end points, to date their validity remains to be proved. Therefore a valid imaging surrogate end point to evaluate therapies for highly morbid conditions such as acute HF, and with the ability to detect improvement of important clinical outcomes, needs to be established.

REFERENCES

1. The Task Force for the Diagnosis and Treatment of Acute and Chronic Heart Failure 2008 of the European Society of Cardiology. ESC guidelines for the diagnosis and treatment of acute and chronic heart failure 2008. Eur Heart J 2008;29:2388–442.
2. 2005 Writing Committee Members. 2009 Focused Update incorporated into the ACC/AHA 2005 Guidelines for the diagnosis and management of heart failure in adults: a report of the American College of Cardiology Foundation/American Heart Association task force on practice guidelines: developed in collaboration with the International Society for Heart and Lung Transplantation. Circulation 2009; 119:e391–479.

3. Rosamond W, Flegal K, Furie K, et al. Heart disease and stroke statistics—2008 update: a report from the American Heart Association Statistics Committee and Stroke Statistics Subcommittee. Circulation 2008;117(4):e25–146.

4. Metra M, Eichhorn E, Abraham WT, et al. Effects of low-dose oral enoximone administration on mortality, morbidity, and exercise capacity in patients with advanced heart failure: the randomized, double-blind, placebo-controlled, parallel group ESSENTIAL trials. Eur Heart J 2009;30(24):3015–26.

5. Felker GM, Pang PS, Adams KF, et al. Clinical trials of pharmacological therapies in acute heart failure syndromes: lessons learned and directions forward. Circ Heart Fail 2010;3(2):314–25.

6. Allen LA, Hernandez AF, O'Connor CM, et al. End points for clinical trials in acute heart failure syndromes. J Am Coll Cardiol 2009;53(24):2248–58.

7. Rector TS, Kubo SH, Cohn JN. Patients' self-assessment of their congestive heart failure: content, reliability and validity of a new measure, the Minnesota Living with Heart Failure questionnaire. Heart Fail 1987;3:198–209.

8. Cohn JN, Goldstein SO, Greenberg BH, et al. A dose-dependent increase in mortality with vesnarinone among patients with severe heart failure. N Engl J Med 1998;339:1810–6.

9. Cohn JN, Tognoni G. A randomized trial of the angiotensin-receptor blocker valsartan in chronic heart failure. N Engl J Med 2001;345:1667–75.

10. Rector TS, Tschumperlin LK, Kubo SH, et al. Use of the living with heart failure questionnaire to ascertain patients' perspectives on improvement in quality of life versus risk of drug-induced death. J Card Fail 1995;1:201–6.

11. Atkinson AJ, Colburn WA, DeGruttola VG, et al. Biomarkers and surrogate endpoints: preferred definitions and conceptual framework. Clin Pharmacol Ther 2001;69(3):89–95.

12. Henderson JA, Smith JJ. Realizing the potential for biomarkers in imaging: background and legal basis. Food Drug Law J 2005;60:511–24.

13. Braunwald E. Biomarkers in heart failure. N Engl J Med 2008;358(20):2148–59.

14. Lesko LJ, Atkinson AJ Jr. Use of biomarkers and surrogate endpoints in drug development and regulatory decision making: criteria, validation, strategies. Annu Rev Pharmacol Toxicol 2001;41:347–66.

15. Lipicky RJ, Packer M. Role of surrogate end points in the evaluation of drugs for heart failure. J Am Coll Cardiol 1993;22:179A–84A.

16. Anand IS, Florea VG, Fisher L. Surrogate end points in heart failure. J Am Coll Cardiol 2002;39(9):1414–21.

17. Prentice RL. Surrogate endpoints in clinical trials: definition and operational criteria. Stat Med 1989;8:431–40.

18. Nagueh SF, Kopelen HA, Zoghbi WA. Relation of mean right atrial pressure to echocardiographic and Doppler parameters of right atrial and right ventricular function. Circulation 1996;93:1160–9.

19. Franklin KM, Aurigemma GP. Prognosis in diastolic heart failure. Prog Cardiovasc Dis 2005;47:333–9.

20. Aurigemma GP, Gottdiener JS, Shemanskii L, et al. Predictive value of systolic and diastolic function for incident congestive heart failure in the elderly: the Cardiovascular Health Study. J Am Coll Cardiol 2001;37:1042–8.

21. Pinamonti B, Zecchin M, Di Lenarda A, et al. Persistence of restrictive left ventricular filling pattern in dilated cardiomyopathy: an ominous prognostic sign. J Am Coll Cardiol 1997;29:604–12.

22. Dini FL, Dell' Anna R, Micheli A, et al. Impact of blunted pulmonary venous flow on the outcome of patients with left ventricular systolic dysfunction secondary to either ischemic or idiopathic dilated cardiomyopathy. Am J Cardiol 2000;85:1455–60.

23. Takemoto Y, Barnes ME, Seward JB, et al. Usefulness of left atrial volume in predicting first congestive heart failure in patients > or = 65 years of age with well-preserved left ventricular systolic function. Am J Cardiol 2005;96:832–6.

24. Dokainish H, Zoghbi WA, Lakkis NM, et al. Comparative accuracy of B-type natriuretic peptide and tissue Doppler echocardiography in the diagnosis of congestive heart failure. Am J Cardiol 2004;93:1130–5.

25. Wong M, Johnson G, Shabetai R, et al. Echocardiographic variables as prognostic indicators and therapeutic monitors in chronic congestive heart failure. Veterans Affairs cooperative studies V-HeFT I and II. Circulation 1993;87:VI65–70.

26. St. John Sutton M, Pfeffer MA, Plappert T, et al. Quantitative two-dimensional echocardiographic measurements are major predictors of adverse cardiovascular events after acute myocardial infarction. The protective effects of captopril. Circulation 1994;89:68–75.

27. St. John Sutton M, Pfeffer MA, Moye L, et al. Cardiovascular death and left ventricular remodeling two years after myocardial infarction: baseline predictors and impact of long-term use of captopril: information from the Survival And Ventricular Enlargement (SAVE) trial. Circulation 1997;96:3294–9.

28. Doughty RN, Whalley GA, Gamble G, et al. Left ventricular remodeling with carvedilol in patients with congestive heart failure due to ischemic heart disease. Australia-New Zealand Heart Failure Research Collaborative Group. J Am Coll Cardiol 1997;29:1060–6.

29. Doughty RN, Whalley GA, Walsh H, et al. Effects of carvedilol on left ventricular remodeling in patients following acute myocardial infarction: the

CAPRICORN echo substudy. Circulation 2004; 109(2):201–6.

30. Greenberg B, Quinones MA, Koilpillai C, et al. Effects of long-term enalapril therapy on cardiac structure and function in patients with left ventricular dysfunction. Results of the SOLVD echocardiography substudy. Circulation 1995;91:2573–81.

31. Groenning BA, Nilsson JC, Sondergaard L, et al. Anti-remodeling effects on the left ventricle during beta-blockade with metoprolol in the treatment of chronic heart failure. J Am Coll Cardiol 2000;36:2072–80.

32. Cintron G, Johnson G, Francis G, et al. Prognostic significance of serial changes in left ventricular ejection fraction in patients with congestive heart failure. Circulation 1993;87:VI17–23.

33. Packer M, Carver JR, Rodeheffer RJ, et al. Effect of oral milrinone on mortality in severe chronic heart failure. N Engl J Med 1991;325:1468–75.

34. McKelvie RS, Yusuf S, Pericak D, et al. Comparison of candesartan, enalapril, and their combination in congestive heart failure: randomized evaluation of strategies for left ventricular dysfunction (RESOLVD) pilot study. Circulation 1999;100:1056–64.

35. Tei C, Ling LH, Hodge DO, et al. New index of combined systolic and diastolic myocardial performance: a simple and reproducible measure of cardiac function—a study in normals and dilated cardiomyopathy. J Cardiol 1995;26:357–66.

36. Dujardin KS, Tei T, Yeo TC, et al. Prognostic value of a Doppler index combining systolic and diastolic performance in idiopathic-dilated cardiomyopathy. Am J Cardiol 1998;82:1071–6.

37. Mikkelsen KV, Moller JE, Bie P, et al. Tei index and neurohormonal activation in patients with incident heart failure: serial changes and prognostic value. Eur J Heart Fail 2006;8:599–608.

38. Cooper RS, Simmons BE, Castaner A, et al. Left ventricular hypertrophy is associated with worse survival independent of ventricular function and number of coronary arteries severely narrowed. Am J Cardiol 1990;65:441–5.

39. Quinones MA, Breenberg BH, Kopelen HA, et al, for the SOLVD Investigators. Echocardiographic predictors of clinical outcomes in patients with left ventricular dysfunction enrolled in the SOLVD registry and trials: significance of left ventricular hypertrophy. J Am Coll Cardiol 2005;35:1237–44.

40. Devereux RB, de Simone G, Ganau A, et al. Left ventricular hypertrophy and geometric remodeling in hypertension: stimuli, functional consequences and prognostic implications. J Hypertens 1994;12:S117–27.

41. Rossi A, Luigi Temporelli P, Quintana M, et al, on behalf of the MeRGE Heart Failure Collaborators. Independent relationship of left atrial size and mortality in patients with heart failure: an individual patient meta-analysis of longitudinal data (MeRGE Heart Failure). Eur J Heart Fail 2009;11:929–36. DOI:10.1093/eurjhf/hfp112.

42. Larose E, Ganz P, Reynolds HG, et al. Right ventricular dysfunction assessed by cardiovascular magnetic resonance imaging predicts poor prognosis late after myocardial infarction. J Am Coll Cardiol 2007;49:855–62.

43. Gulati VK, Katz WE, Follansbee WP, et al. Mitral annular descent velocity by tissue Doppler echocardiography as an index of global left ventricular function. Am J Cardiol 1996;77:979–84.

44. Yip G, Wang M, Zhang Y, et al. Left ventricular long axis function in diastolic heart failure is reduced in both diastole and systole: time for a redefinition? Heart 2002;87:121–5.

45. Troughton RW, Prior DL, Frampton CM, et al. Usefulness of tissue Doppler and color M-mode indexes of left ventricular diastolic function in predicting outcomes in systolic left ventricular heart failure (from the ADEPT study). Am J Cardiol 2005;96:257–62.

46. Bello D, Fieno DS, Kim RJ, et al. Infarct morphology identifies patients with substrate for sustained ventricular tachycardia. J Am Coll Cardiol 2005;45:1104–8.

47. Yan AT, Shayne AJ, Brown KA, et al. Characterization of the peri-infarct zone by contrast-enhanced cardiac magnetic resonance imaging is a powerful predictor of post-myocardial infarction mortality. Circulation 2006;114:32–9.

48. Schmidt A, Azevedo CF, Cheng A, et al. Infarct tissue heterogeneity by magnetic resonance imaging identifies enhanced cardiac arrhythmia susceptibility in patients with left ventricular dysfunction. Circulation 2007;115:2006–14.

49. Borges-Neto S, Shaw LK, Tuttle RH, et al. Incremental prognostic power of single-photon emission computed tomographic myocardial perfusion imaging in patients with known or suspected coronary artery disease. Am J Cardiol 2005;95:182–8.

50. van der Burg AE, Bax JJ, Boersma E, et al. Impact of viability, ischemia, scar tissue, and revascularization on outcome after aborted sudden death. Circulation 2003;108:1954–9.

51. Piccini JP, Horton JR, Shaw LK, et al. Single-photon emission computed tomography myocardial perfusion defects are associated with an increased risk of all-cause death, cardiovascular death, and sudden cardiac death. Circ Cardiovasc Imaging 2008;1:180–8.

52. Mehta SR, Eikelboom JW, Natarajan MK, et al. Impact of right ventricular involvement on mortality and morbidity in patients with inferior myocardial infarction. J Am Coll Cardiol 2001;37(1):37–43.

53. Stolen KQ, Kemppainen J, Kalliokoski KK, et al. Myocardial perfusion reserve and peripheral endothelial function in patients with idiopathic dilated cardiomyopathy. Am J Cardiol 2004;93:64–8.

54. Neglia D, Michelassi C, Trivieri MG, et al. Prognostic role of myocardial blood flow impairment in idiopathic left ventricular dysfunction. Circulation 2002; 105:186–93.

55. Wu KC, Zerhouni EA, Judd RM, et al. Prognostic significance of microvascular obstruction by magnetic resonance imaging in patients with acute myocardial infarction. Circulation 1998;97:765–72.

56. Kwong RY, Chan AK, Brown KA, et al. Impact of unrecognized myocardial scar detected by cardiac magnetic resonance imaging on event-free survival in patients presenting with signs or symptoms of coronary artery disease. Circulation 2006;113: 2733–43.

57. Assomull RG, Prasad SK, Lyne J, et al. Cardiovascular magnetic resonance, fibrosis, and prognosis in dilated cardiomyopathy. J Am Coll Cardiol 2006; 48:1977–85.

58. Wu KC, Weiss RG, Thiemann DR, et al. Late gadolinium enhancement by cardiovascular magnetic resonance heralds an adverse prognosis in nonischemic cardiomyopathy. J Am Coll Cardiol 2008; 51:2414–21.

59. Nazarian S, Bluemke DA, Lardo AC, et al. Magnetic resonance assessment of the substrate for inducible ventricular tachycardia in nonischemic cardiomyopathy. Circulation 2005;112:2821–5.

60. Borges-Neto S. LBCT II. Presented at: Heart Failure Society of America 13th Annual Scientific Meeting. Heart Failure Society News Volume 11, Number 2, December 2009. Boston, September 13-16, 2009.

61. Agostini D, Verberne HJ, Burchert W, et al. I-123-mIBG myocardial imaging for assessment of risk for a major cardiac event in heart failure patients: insights from a retrospective European multicenter study. Eur J Nucl Med Mol Imaging 2008;35:535–46.

62. Nakata T, Wakabayashi T, Kyuma M, et al. Prognostic implications of an initial loss of cardiac meta-iodobenzylguanidine uptake and diabetes mellitus in patients with left ventricular dysfunction. J Card Fail 2003;9(2):113–21.

63. Paul M, Schäfers M, Kies P, et al. Impact of sympathetic innervation on recurrent life-threatening arrhythmias in the follow-up of patients with idiopathic ventricular fibrillation. Eur J Nucl Med Mol Imaging 2006;33(8):866–70.

64. Yamada T, Shimonagata T, Fukunami M, et al. Comparison of the prognostic value of cardiac iodine-123 metaiodobenzylguanidine imaging and heart rate variability in patients with chronic heart failure: a prospective study. J Am Coll Cardiol 2003;41:231–8.

65. Jacobson AF, Senior R, Cerqueira MD, et al. Myocardial iodine-123 meta-iodobenzylguanidine imaging and cardiac events in heart failure results of the prospective ADMIRE-HF (AdreView Myocardial Imaging for Risk Evaluation in Heart Failure) Study. J Am Coll Cardiol 2010;55:2212–21.

66. Allman KC, Shaw LJ, Hachamovitch R, et al. Myocardial viability testing and impact of revascularization on prognosis in patients with coronary artery disease and left ventricular dysfunction: a meta-analysis. J Am Coll Cardiol 2002;39(7):1151–8.

Cardiorenal Syndrome Clinical Trial End Points

Robert J. Mentz, MD[a],*, Christopher M. O'Connor, MD[b]

KEYWORDS

- Heart failure • Cardiorenal syndrome • Clinical trials
- End points

Acute heart failure syndromes (AHFS) encompass a heterogeneous group of clinical entities involving new or worsening signs or symptoms of heart failure (HF) resulting in hospitalization. AHFS are the leading cause of hospitalization for persons more than 65 years of age with more than 1 million hospitalizations annually in the United States.[1] Renal impairment is common in all categories of HF irrespective of ejection fraction or overt symptoms,[2,3] and it serves as an independent risk factor for morbidity and mortality.[4] Only recently has a framework for this dual organ dysfunction termed cardiorenal syndrome (CRS) been offered to clinicians, and a consensus definition has not been definitively established. Ronco and colleagues[5] outline 4 categories of CRS that stress the complex and bidirectional interplay between the failing heart and kidney in both the acute and chronic disease states. The underlying pathophysiology of CRS is incompletely understood but likely involves variable contributions in different patients of central venous congestion, neurohormonal and renal sympathetic activity, oxidative stress, and anemia, plus additional undefined mechanisms.[6] Because of the lack of consensus definitions, limited understanding of the pathophysiology and high mortality of CRS, patients with renal dysfunction have largely been excluded from HF trials. Consequently, the appropriate management for patients with CRS is unknown even with respect to medicines that are well validated and evidence based for the general HF population (eg, β-blockers and angiotensin-converting enzyme inhibitors). Some data support that those with renal dysfunction may be the group to benefit the most from HF therapies.[7] The heterogeneity of AHFS, but the commonality of CRS, makes this patient population a key target for investigation of novel therapies.

Recent clinical trials investigating novel HF therapies with potential effects on CRS have failed to show benefit with respect to key end points.[8–10] Possible explanations for these recent disappointments include the lack of understanding of underlying pathophysiology and the heterogeneity of the AHFS patient population, compounded by the lack of standardized clinical trial end points.[11,12] The International AHFS Working Group has offered a framework for future research in AHFS that emphasizes efficacy and safety with potential end points ranging from patient-centered criteria, index hospitalization data, and post-discharge events to composite end points, but consensus has yet to be established.[13–15] This article reviews the end points evaluated in several key clinical trials of CRS and synthesizes recent discussions about the appropriateness of AHFS end points, specifically with respect to CRS.

DEFINING CARDIORENAL SYNDROME FOR CLINICAL TRIALS

Given that the early AHFS trials excluded patients with renal dysfunction, much of the initial clinical data on those with acute CRS comes from

Financial disclosures: RJM, none; CMO, none.
[a] Division of Cardiology, Department of Medicine, Duke University Medical Center, 2301 Erwin Road, Durham, NC 27705, USA
[b] Division of Cardiology, Duke University Medical Center, DUMC 3356, Durham, NC 27710, USA
* Corresponding author.
E-mail address: robert.mentz@duke.edu

Heart Failure Clin 7 (2011) 519–528
doi:10.1016/j.hfc.2011.06.012

retrospective analyses. Worsening renal function (WRF) during hospitalization for AHFS represents the best-characterized population of patients with CRS. Although initial studies used a variety of cutoffs to characterize WRF, a creatinine increase greater than or equal to 0.3 mg/dL during hospitalization is now most commonly used, because this provides the maximum sensitivity and specificity for outcomes data.[16–20] As reviewed previously, WRF has been associated with an increased length of stay, in-hospital complication rate, cost, and mortality to 5 years.[21] However, not all studies support an association between WRF and worse outcome,[22,23] so a consensus WRF definition has not been universally accepted to characterize CRS. Furthermore, although WRF occurs in approximately 30% of AHFS admissions,[21] this classification only captures 1 subgroup of patients with acute CRS. For instance, those with acute kidney injury (AKI) on admission would not be included in this category if their creatinine did not subsequently increase to greater than or equal to 0.3 mg/dL during hospitalization. Those with AKI could be the subset of patients with CRS at highest risk and potentially could receive the greatest benefit from novel therapies. Further complicating standardization, the use of creatinine fluctuation likely does not capture the complexity of cardiorenal interactions given that creatinine may take days to become increased following a renal insult. Novel biomarkers such as serum neutrophil gelatinase-associated lipocalin (NGAL), urine interleukin (IL)-18, and kidney injury molecule-1 (KIM-1) may allow for earlier detection of CRS and could offer more representative markers of renal dysfunction.[24] Given the limitations of using WRF and creatinine, further investigation of novel biomarkers as well as alternative renal function assessments (eg, estimated glomerular filtration rate [eGFR] decrease by $\geq$25%) are critical to standardize acute CRS definitions. In the meantime, we propose that future CRS trials should attempt to capture a broader spectrum of acute CRS including patients with WRF and acute renal failure using eGFR at a minimum, and ideally also with novel biomarkers.

In comparison with acute CRS, there are even fewer data on those with chronic CRS given creatinine cutoffs as exclusion criteria in most HF trials. At least moderate (stage III) chronic kidney disease (CKD), defined as an eGFR less than 60 mL/min/1.73 m^2, is present in up to 60% of patients with HF.[21] This criterion offers a starting point to investigate chronic CRS. While waiting for future consensus definitions, we propose that trials evaluating chronic CRS should include patients with at least moderate CKD and then perform analyses based on the progressive stages of CKD. Subgroup analyses by the different eGFR cutoffs could provide insight into those patients at different points in the spectrum of CRS.

END POINTS IN CLINICAL TRIALS OF CARDIORENAL SYNDROME
VMAC – Nesiritide: Dyspnea and Hemodynamics

The history of nesiritide offers a framework for discussion on initial clinical trial end points in CRS. Receiving US Food and Drug Administration (FDA) approval in 2001, nesiritide, a recombinant analogue of human brain natriuretic peptide, was the last novel agent approved for AHFS. Although the main effect of nesiritide is vasodilation, early work supported a pathophysiologic potential for renal protective effects (eg, increased glomerular filtration rate [GFR], suppression of the renin-angiotensin-aldosterone axis).[25] Initial nesiritide trials were small, randomized clinical trials (n = 103 and 127) that indicated short-term improvements (assessment at 1–24 hours) in pulmonary capillary wedge pressure (PCWP), global clinical status, and dyspnea.[26,27] Nesiritide may have renal protective effects but these were not investigated in initial clinical trials.

Following these trials, the VMAC (Vasodilation in the Management of Acute Congestive Heart Failure) study in 2002 was a large, multicenter, randomized, double-blind trial of 489 patients with AHFS randomized to nesiritide, nitroglycerin, or placebo in addition to standard care.[28] The trial showed that nesiritide significantly improved the primary end points of PCWP and dyspnea (Likert scale) as seen in earlier studies. Nesiritide did not improve 30-day rehospitalization and mortality. With regard to renal function end points, the investigators only reported that "through 30 days, there were no significant differences in the frequency of serious adverse events or pattern of changes in serum creatinine."

VMAC's lack of discussion on a CRS end point until a retrospective follow-up article allowed several meta-analyses to highlight potential safety concerns. Although the initial VMAC trial was not powered for statistical comparison of renal dysfunction, Butler and colleagues[29] performed a retrospective review of the small number of patients (n = 60) with renal insufficiency (RI; creatinine $\geq$2.0 mg/dL) compared with those without RI for end points of efficacy and safety. Renal function was preserved in patients with RI who received nesiritide, and there was no significant difference in serious adverse events, 30-day readmission/death, or 6-month mortality. However, several meta-analyses in 2005 of data from VMAC and other small randomized trials of nesiritide raised the hypotheses that nesiritide may worsen renal function[30] and decrease survival at 30 days.[31] These meta-analyses resulted in a substantial reduction in the use of nesiritide.[32] The history of nesiritide shows how a medication with pathophysiologic potential for renal protective effects can be largely sidelined from clinical use by retrospective analyses when trials are not designed to evaluate the role of CRS. A landmark nesiritide trial is discussed later.

Further review of the primary end points used in VMAC provides insight into designing CRS clinical trials. The VMAC study's primary end point of dyspnea has been controversial. VMAC was the first randomized AHFS clinical trial to show a positive finding using a clinical end point (ie, patient-perceived dyspnea). This patient-centered outcome seems relevant because dyspnea is the symptom that brings most patients with AHFS to medical attention. Teerlink[33] writes that dyspnea improvement is one of the most important standards for measuring efficacy of therapy in AHFS. Moreover, for a drug to receive FDA approval, it must either improve symptoms or clinical outcomes for a particular disease.[34] However, evaluation of dyspnea does not include objective data, lacks standardization, and largely improves regardless of intervention.[12]

West and colleagues[34] recently reviewed the literature on dyspnea in AHFS. They discuss the use of the Likert scale and Visual Analog Scale (VAS) in AHFS trials. Although both instruments have shortcomings (eg, intersubject variability with VAS), the investigators provide a starting point for future trials to improve standardization and reproducibility. For example, they describe characterizing the minimal clinically important difference (MCID) for these scales in AHFS to pinpoint the smallest improvement in scores that patients perceive as beneficial. They also describe use of the Dyspnea Severity Score (DSS) to standardize dyspnea scores during various measures including position variation, oxygen removal, and ambulation. With respect to CRS trials, we support a dyspnea efficacy end point that incorporates these techniques for standardization.

The use of a hemodynamic end point for clinical outcomes has also been contentious. The discordance between hemodynamic data and hard end points in VMAC calls into question the use of these parameters as surrogates for efficacy. An ideal surrogate should have a strong and consistent relationship with outcome (including a pathophysiologic as well as a statistical relationship) that is replicated in a variety of different populations.[35] Although

reducing PCWP has previously been correlated with symptomatic improvement and prognostic importance,[36,37] several trials in the 1990s showed that medications causing significant hemodynamic improvements may increase mortality (eg, milrinone, vesnarinone, epoprostenol).[38–40] Moreover, hemodynamic data have not always been successful in guiding dose selection in new AHFS drug development (eg, tezosentan).[12] Alternatively, as Anand and colleagues[35] describe, all the current drugs approved for HF treatments have long-term beneficial hemodynamic effects. Therefore, although hemodynamic data alone should not commonly be used as a CRS primary end point, such data do provide important information regarding underlying pathophysiology. The aftereffects of VMAC on nesiritide use show the importance of investigating CRS end points a priori and critically appraising end point selection, particularly with respect to nonvalidated surrogates.

ESCAPE – Pulmonary Artery Catheterization: Hemodynamics, Days Alive and Out of Hospital

The ESCAPE (Evaluation Study of Congestive Heart Failure and Pulmonary Artery [PA] Catheterization Effectiveness) trial provided further insight into hemodynamic end points, raised a key hypothesis about WRF in CRS, and introduced a novel composite end point for CRS trials.[22,41] The ESCAPE trial was a multicenter, randomized controlled trial (n = 433) evaluating the use of PA catheter-guided therapy compared with treatment based on clinical assessment alone with regard to the primary end point of days alive and out of hospital at 6 months. The treatment goal of those managed with PA catheters was to target a PCWP less than or equal to 15 mm Hg and right atrial pressure (RAP) less than or equal to 8 mm Hg. Other secondary end points included quality of life, exercise capacity, biomarker data, and echocardiographic changes. Patients with a creatinine more than 3.5 mg/dL were excluded from the trial. Treatment in both groups led to substantial reductions in AHFS signs and symptoms and there was no difference between the treatment strategies with respect to the primary end point of days alive and out of hospital or with regard to the secondary end points.

Nohria and colleagues[22] performed a retrospective review of the ESCAPE data to characterize the pathophysiology and impact of renal dysfunction in patients admitted with AHFS. First, with respect to hemodynamics, they found no correlation between baseline hemodynamics or changes in hemodynamics and WRF. Only RAP correlated weakly with baseline renal function. These data further support concerns about the use of isolated hemodynamic measurements as a target in CRS. Improving hemodynamics without affecting other components of the CRS pathophysiologic cascade should not be expected to necessarily improve outcomes. Second, although baseline and discharge RI were associated with an increased risk of death and death or rehospitalization at 6 months, WRF was not associated with worse outcomes. These data raised a new hypothesis about the underlying pathophysiology of CRS and how CRS should be investigated in clinical trials. Nohria and colleagues[22] write that "perhaps [WRF] is inevitable in these patients with risk factors such as hypertension and diabetes and should be viewed as a marker of intrinsic kidney disease rather than a signal to limit adequate diuresis and symptom resolution." This is further substantiated by the recent DOSE (Diuretic Optimization Strategies Evaluation) study, in which investigators found that the effects of high-dose furosemide on worsening renal function in AHFS were transient and not associated with worse outcome at 60 days.[23] Not only is it possible that WRF may not be the most appropriate surrogate for evaluation of CRS end points but also the entire hypothesis of the significance of acute CRS (as is currently defined) is in doubt. Future investigation is needed to confirm these observations and provide insight into appropriate renal function parameters or alternative surrogates for acute CRS.

One of the primary end points applicable to CRS that was evaluated in ESCAPE is days alive and out of hospital. Some of the benefits of this composite include its ability to capture the effects of morbidity and mortality into a single end point. Unlike analyses that are merely concerned with the time to the first event, days alive and out of hospital captures the burden of multiple hospitalizations and identifies patients who may initially do poorly but ultimately receive long-term benefit.[42] This may be critical in trials of CRS because mortality benefits are investigated while incorporating the morbidity associated with the increased readmission rate. Given the interdependence between renal and cardiac dysfunction, composite end points may be the best technique to capture the balance between multisystem dysfunction. However, because typically more than one-third of patients have no events at the time of follow-up, outcomes may be skewed with many patients receiving perfect scores. These effects increase the complexity of outcome interpretation and require less powerful, nonparametric techniques for data analysis.[42] More powerful data analysis methods are possible by adjusting for quality of

life, but there is no standard or validated way to adjust the balance between longevity and quality of life. Moreover, even if days hospitalized is rated as badly as days lost because of death, hospitalization ultimately has little net impact compared with death because the number of days is much fewer. Additional criticisms of this end point include that a long index length of stay may decrease statistical power, initial sample size calculations may be unreliable, and the duration of follow-up has a strong impact on outcome.[12,42] An end point of days alive and out of hospital provides some features that are enticing as a CRS end point, but these key criticisms limit universal application.

EVEREST – Tolvaptan: Composites End points, Global Clinical Status, Weight Loss

The EVEREST (Efficacy of Vasopressin Antagonism in Heart Failure Outcome Study with Tolvaptan) trials used end points including composites, and global clinical status as well as surrogates such as weight loss.[8,43] The EVEREST trials investigated the use of tolvaptan, an oral vasopressin V2-receptor antagonist, on short-term clinical status as well as long-term outcome in 2 randomized, controlled trials of more than 4000 patients with AHFS. The primary end point of the clinical status trial was the composite end point of global clinical status (via a 100-point VAS) and weight loss at 7 days or discharge if earlier. Rank sum analysis showed a statistically significant improvement of the primary composite end point with tolvaptan versus placebo, but there was no difference in global clinical status. With regard to renal end points, serum urea nitrogen and creatinine were collected at day 1, 7, and discharge. Creatinine increased slightly more in the tolvaptan group than in the placebo group but there was no excess of renal failure. The dual primary end point for the outcome trial was all-cause mortality (superiority and noninferiority) and cardiovascular (CV) death or HF hospitalization. During a median follow-up of more than 9 months, there was no significant difference between tolvaptan and placebo with respect to these end points.

Composite end points such as that used in the EVEREST clinical status trial have both positive and negative aspects to keep in perspective. Composite end points are designed to combine components of AHFS into a single integrated measure.[12] One key benefit of a composite end point is the potential for a higher event rate and, as long as the treatment has the ability to affect all the components of the composite, then the trial's sample size can be smaller.[44] Composite end points that are appropriately selected can be helpful in CRS trials in which event rates may be lower with the use of current evidence-based medical regimens. This statistical efficiency could also allow for sufficient sample sizes to evaluate differential benefits in subgroups of CRS; this could represent a method to investigate the heterogeneity of AHFS. Composite end points may have the benefit of potentially improving power and decreasing sample size, but the ability to detect benefit can be diluted by the inclusion of an outcome for which treatment exhibits no effect. A recent review of composite outcomes in clinical trials indicates that discordance between components is common.[45] Furthermore, if the treatment effect is different on the constituents of the composite, then the results can be difficult to interpret. For instance, although the primary end point in the EVEREST clinical status trial was positive, it was driven completely by the weight loss component with no improvement in global clinical status. Composite results must not be misinterpreted as necessarily indicating benefit for all the components of the end point. Previous literature has supported using each component of the composite as a secondary end point, as seen in EVEREST, to reduce this ambiguity.[45] The appropriate balance between the use of composite end points to allow demonstration of efficacy and the use of primary end points with clear clinical applicability for AHFS is currently debated.[14]

Additional discussions on EVEREST pertain to the use of weight loss and global clinical status end points. The use of a weight loss end point seems beneficial because congestion is responsible for the presentation of most patients with AHFS and fluid removal with weight loss would be expected to be the natural progression of treatment. However, data from the Acute Decompensated Heart Failure National Registry (ADHERE) indicate that 50% of patients do not experience significant body weight reduction but are considered to be ready for discharge,[46] and recent data from implantable hemodynamic monitors suggest that the relationship with total body volume retention may be more complex than previously believed.[47] The recent UNLOAD study evaluating ultrafiltration in AHFS also used the coprimary end point of weight loss at 48 hours (along with dyspnea).[9] Similar results were observed to those of EVEREST, in which the change in weight loss and not symptoms drove the end point. Taken together, these data indicate that a better understanding of the role of volume and weight loss, along with further end point validation, are required before accepting weight loss as a CRS trial end point. Vigilance is needed to prevent fluid

status from becoming a red herring in CRS trials, as seen with a hemodynamic end point.

Although neither weight loss nor global clinical status have been validated as end points in AHFS, it could be argued that the global clinical status or general well-being of patients captures the more significant domain. When using composite outcomes to capture effect, it must be remembered that all outcomes are not perceived equally. This concept leads to considerations of weighting components of the composite to capture the proportional significance to the patient's clinical experience (eg, a global ranking approach), as is further expounded on later.

The EVEREST outcome trial used dual primary end points to investigate hard end point data. The coprimary end points of death and HF hospitalization capture both morbidity and mortality effects similar to days alive and out of hospital. However, use of more than 1 primary end point requires that the potential for type I error (ie, false positive) is allocated to multiple end points in comparison with composite end points that are integrated into 1 measure. Coprimary end points may require a larger sample size than composites. Nonetheless, when investigating evidence of treatment effect on multiple outcome measures, coprimary end points serve as the gold standard. To date, coprimary end points in HF trials typically have included CV mortality or hospitalization. We propose that because CRS includes both renal and cardiac dysfunction, trial end points should incorporate coprimary end points targeting both organ systems.

Decisions about the appropriate mortality and hospitalization end points require careful consideration when designing CRS trials. Mortality is an important AHFS trial end point given the substantial risk of death and desire for new therapies to show a survival advantage. The use of all-cause mortality versus disease-specific mortality has been debated. Although all-cause mortality has a higher overall event rate and does not require adjudication, it can diminish a study's power because non–disease-specific deaths may be less likely to benefit from a novel HF therapy.[12] Moreover, the heterogeneity of the AHFS population, compounded by the limited timeframe in which novel therapies are tested during hospitalization, complicate the ability to detect long-term benefit. Perhaps it is not reasonable to expect long-term mortality benefit from a limited-duration therapy, and alternative CRS end points may be more appropriate. The inclusion of hospitalizations is not straightforward either. Although the morbidity associated with repeat hospitalizations is evident, early hospitalization may not necessarily be a negative characteristic if it reflects close outpatient monitoring of patients and attempts at early intervention.[48] There are also substantial regional differences in patterns of admission and length of stay, which can complicate applicability of different studies. Ideally, future CRS trials should mirror EVEREST by incorporating coprimary end points that capture the multiplicity of hard outcomes, but further study is needed to clarify the appropriate blend for CRS.

The EVEREST trial also included both superiority and noninferiority as end points with respect to all-cause mortality, which enabled the authors to indicate that tolvaptan may not offer survival advantages compared with current therapy but it can improve clinical parameters such as dyspnea and weight loss with a reasonable safety profile (ie, no worse than standard care). In effect, this enabled the drug to remain on the market for patients whose fluid and electrolytes or renal function may limit conventional therapies; it prevented tolvaptan from completely experiencing the post-trial fate as seen with nesiritide after VMAC. Future trials are needed to validate this noninferiority approach for CRS.

PROTECT – Rolofylline: a Trichotomous Composite End point, Dyspnea, Worsening HF

The recent PROTECT study used a trichotomous composite end point to evaluate a novel therapy in CRS.[10] Early studies with adenosine antagonists supported their ability to enhance diuresis while maintaining or improving renal function.[49,50] The PROTECT study randomized more than 2000 patients with AHFS and impaired renal function (creatinine clearance of 20–80 mL/min) to rolofylline versus placebo within 24 hours of hospitalization for up to 3 days with 180-day follow-up. PROTECT is therefore one of the largest trials to date that specifically investigated CRS and it includes the widest spectrum of renal dysfunction in an AHFS trial. The primary end point was treatment success, failure or no change where success was defined as improvement in dyspnea (Likert scale at 24 and 48 hours) in the absence of any treatment failure including death (ie, death or HF readmission through 7 days), worsening of HF requiring rescue therapy (ie, increased intravenous or mechanical therapy for HF), and end-organ damage with persistent renal impairment (creatinine increase ≥ 0.3 mg/dL during hospitalization and confirmed at day 7 and 14 or initiation of dialysis). The investigators used a new definition for persistent renal impairment that had not previously been clinically investigated. Future validation of this definition or an alternative is critical to the

CRS clinical trial enterprise. Secondary end points captured the components of the composite, including persistent renal impairment and the 60-day rate of death or readmission for CV or renal causes. Rolofylline did not provide benefit with respect to any of these end points. Although significantly more patients in the rolofylline group showed improvement in dyspnea compared with placebo, an excess of patients with persistent renal impairment in the rolofylline group counterbalanced any benefit.

The use of a trichotomous end point such as that of PROTECT was designed to provide a single quantitative analysis of the full spectrum of treatment effects.[51] Although the trial's end point of success versus failure reduces some of the complexity inherent in composite analysis, there are several potential downsides to this approach. When looking at the constituents of the primary composite end point in PROTECT, an improvement in dyspnea was the only positive attribute included. In contrast, failure criteria included mortality, rehospitalization, increased HF therapy, and WRF. The study design set the bar high for rolofylline to demonstrate superiority. For instance, take 2 patients randomized to rolofylline, – 1 who is subsequently hospitalized multiple times during the first 60 days and 1 who has an increase in creatinine by 0.3 mg/dL that persists. Even if both of these patients ultimately live longer than if they had received placebo, then, regardless of the clinical benefit, both of these patients would be counted as treatment failures. In addition, concluding that rolofylline does not afford clinical efficacy in CRS because of a lack of benefit for creatinine increase at 7 and 14 days may be incorrect. This end point has never been validated and data from ESCAPE and DOSE directly refute the use of a WRF end point.[22,23] Had rolofylline resulted in benefit for all the end points, there would have been a broad application for the drug. However, benefit was not observed in all patients admitted with AHFS and RI, which is consistent with the heterogeneity that typifies the AHFS population. Perhaps future subgroup analyses of those with different types of CRS will reveal certain patients who may benefit from rolofylline. Although a trichotomous end point can reduce the complexity of composites, identification of the specific constituents of such an end point that best captures safety and efficacy for CRS requires further investigation.

The observations from pilot studies of adenosine antagonists provide key considerations for designing future trials. The positive results of the rolofylline pilot study[52] followed by the negative phase III trial highlight the critical role of the large-scale clinical trial. The reasons for the lack of benefit in PROTECT are unknown. However, additional adenosine antagonist pilot studies continue to show signs of a positive effect on renal function.[53] Careful analysis of these novel agents is required to determine their potential role (if any) in patients with AHFS. These agents may not show broad efficacy in all patients with AHFS but they may have benefit in certain subgroups of CRS. Clinical trial end points should strive to capture the differential benefit of novel agents in the heterogeneous AHFS population.

A GLOBAL RANK END POINT

The lack of benefit with new AHFS therapies using current end points has led to the proposal for novel approaches such as a global rank end point. As noted earlier for patients receiving tolvaptan, composite end points may not capture the totality of patient and physician experience. Felker and colleagues[54,55] attempted to tackle this problem with a global ranking approach in AHFS trials. A global rank end point ranks all patients based on a prespecified hierarchical ranking of various components of their clinical course.[54] Events such as death or hospitalization as well as quantitative assessments such as dyspnea, quality of life, or biomarker surrogates could be incorporated into outcome analysis. Patients with the worst and earliest outcome would be ranked lowest and patients with less serious events would be ranked sequentially higher. Following the creation of the rank list, the treatment arms can be analyzed with statistical methods to determine the comparative effectiveness.[56] In addition, the use of quantitative assessments such as biomarkers allows for the incorporation of data that may reflect underlying pathophysiology that can be targeted in different patient subgroups. For instance, Felker and Maisel[54] write that biomarker surrogates of myocardial or renal injury may indicate that improvement in congestion only helps those who do not experience untoward end-organ injury. Perhaps biomarkers or other surrogates that reflect differences in pathophysiology of CRS could allow for targeted evaluation of therapeutic efficacy, analogous to the use of tissue markers to provide targeted therapy in different oncologic diseases. Criticisms of a global rank approach include that it may make summarizing the results of trials more difficult and that it could allow a global rank end point to be significant even with individual components that do not show significant differences. Although the latter is an inherent problem in all composite end points, presenting the results of the individual components

allows for a full analysis of efficacy and safety. A global rank end point addresses some of the limitations observed with other methodologies but would require further validation.

ASCEND-HF – Nesiritide: Bridging from Dyspnea to Composite End points

The ASCEND-HF (Acute Study of Clinical Effectiveness of Nesiritide in Decompensated Heart Failure) trial incorporated many of the end points discussed earlier and provides a framework for future CRS trials. As the first mega-trial in AHFS, ASCEND-HF included more than 7000 patients with AHFS randomized to nesiritide infusion for 1 to 7 days.[57] The 2 coprimary end points were patient-assessed dyspnea (Likert scale) at 6 or 24 hours, and a composite of 30-day HF rehospitalization and all-cause mortality. Key secondary end points included 3 composites: (1) persistent or worsening HF and all-cause mortality during the index hospitalization, (2) number of days alive and out of hospital up to 30 days, and (3) CV death and rehospitalization from CV causes up to 30 days. The renal impairment end point in the trial used yet another definition with a greater than or equal to 25% decrease in eGFR at the end of drug infusion, day 10 or discharge, and at day 30. There was no significant difference with nesiritide therapy in any of the trial's endpoints except for increased hypotension. While ASCEND-HF was a neutral trial, its rigorous methodology should focus attention on continued standardization of end points in CRS trials. For instance, the investigators provide a discussion of the implications of differing regulatory views on endpoint selection and data analysis and include prespecified subgroup analyses (eg, women, minorities, patients with preserved systolic function and renal disease).

REGULATORY CONSIDERATIONS

The lack of consensus by regulatory bodies for approval of new drugs further complicates trial design. For instance, the European Medicines Agency (EMEA) prefers the efficacy end point of 30-day mortality, with symptomatic combined with hemodynamic improvement also being adequate.[13] However, the EMEA has not embraced repeat hospitalization or composite end points as used in the United States.[12] The FDA accepts a meaningful clinical benefit that includes symptoms, preservation of renal function, and/or reduction in morbidity/mortality. Hemodynamic measurements can also be part of a primary end point. This substantial variability further clouds study design of international AHFS trials as the interests of licensing authorities, sponsors, and trialists conflict.

SUMMARY

Although the end points in AHFS trials do not approach the standardization of acute coronary syndrome trials, our experience from previous AHFS trials provides guidance for the future. To show a benefit of a novel therapy, not only must the proper patients be selected and the underlying pathophysiology targeted, but there must also be standardized end points that incorporate patient-centered criteria as well as clinically objective efficacy and safety outcomes. CRS trials present further complications given the lack of consensus definitions of CRS and the uncertainty of how best to characterize outcome. The ASCEND-HF study provides useful information on CRS end points having incorporated multiple end points from previous AHFS trials. Nonetheless, the appropriate end points for CRS require further investigation and may be best represented with novel solutions such as a global rank end point.

REFERENCES

1. American Heart Association. 2009 Heart and stroke statistical update. Dallas (TX): American Heart Association; 2009.

2. Hillege HL, Nitsch D, Pfeffer MA, et al. Renal function as a predictor of outcome in a broad spectrum of patients with heart failure. Circulation 2006;113(5):671–8.

3. Dries DL, Exner DV, Domanski MJ, et al. The prognostic implications of renal insufficiency in asymptomatic and symptomatic patients with left ventricular systolic dysfunction. J Am Coll Cardiol 2000;35(3): 681–9.

4. Hillege HL, Girbes AR, de Kam PJ, et al. Renal function, neurohormonal activation, and survival in patients with chronic heart failure. Circulation 2000; 102(2):203–10.

5. Ronco C, Haapio M, House AA, et al. Cardiorenal syndrome. J Am Coll Cardiol 2008;52(19):1527–39.

6. Bock JS, Gottlieb SS. Cardiorenal syndrome: new perspectives. Circulation 2010;121(23):2592–600.

7. Effects of enalapril on mortality in severe congestive heart failure. Results of the Cooperative North Scandinavian Enalapril Survival Study (CONSENSUS). The CONSENSUS Trial Study Group. N Engl J Med 1987;316(23):1429–35.

8. Konstam MA, Gheorghiade M, Burnett JC Jr, et al. Effects of oral tolvaptan in patients hospitalized for worsening heart failure: the EVEREST Outcome Trial. JAMA 2007;297(12):1319–31.

9. Costanzo MR, Guglin ME, Saltzberg MT, et al. Ultrafiltration versus intravenous diuretics for patients hospitalized for acute decompensated heart failure. J Am Coll Cardiol 2007;49(6):675–83.

10. Massie BM, O'Connor CM, Metra M, et al. Rolofylline, an adenosine A1-receptor antagonist, in acute heart failure. N Engl J Med 2010;363(15):1419–28.

11. Gheorghiade M, Pang PS. Acute heart failure syndromes. J Am Coll Cardiol 2009;53(7):557–73.

12. Allen LA, Hernandez AF, O'Connor CM, et al. End points for clinical trials in acute heart failure syndromes. J Am Coll Cardiol 2009;53(24):2248–58.

13. Gheorghiade M, Zannad F, Sopko G, et al. Acute heart failure syndromes: current state and framework for future research. Circulation 2005;112(25): 3958–68.

14. Gheorghiade M, Adams KF, Cleland JG, et al. Phase III clinical trial end points in acute heart failure syndromes: a virtual roundtable with the Acute Heart Failure Syndromes International Working Group. Am Heart J 2009;157(6):957–70.

15. Felker GM, Pang PS, Adams KF, et al. Clinical trials of pharmacological therapies in acute heart failure syndromes: lessons learned and directions forward. Circ Heart Fail 2010;3(2):314–25.

16. Krumholz HM, Chen YT, Vaccarino V, et al. Correlates and impact on outcomes of worsening renal function in patients > or = 65 years of age with heart failure. Am J Cardiol 2000;85(9):1110–3.

17. Butler J, Forman DE, Abraham WT, et al. Relationship between heart failure treatment and development of worsening renal function among hospitalized patients. Am Heart J 2004;147(2):331–8.

18. Forman DE, Butler J, Wang Y, et al. Incidence, predictors at admission, and impact of worsening renal function among patients hospitalized with heart failure. J Am Coll Cardiol 2004;43(1):61–7.

19. Cowie MR, Komajda M, Murray-Thomas T, et al. Prevalence and impact of worsening renal function in patients hospitalized with decompensated heart failure: results of the Prospective Outcomes Study in Heart Failure (POSH). Eur Heart J 2006;27(10): 1216–22.

20. Gottlieb SS, Abraham W, Butler J, et al. The prognostic importance of different definitions of worsening renal function in congestive heart failure. J Card Fail 2002;8(3):136–41.

21. Mentz RJ, Lewis EF. Epidemiology of cardiorenal syndrome. Heart Fail Clin 2010;6(3):333–46.

22. Nohria A, Hasselblad V, Stebbins A, et al. Cardiorenal interactions: insights from the ESCAPE trial. J Am Coll Cardiol 2008;51(13):1268–74.

23. Felker GM, Lee KL, Bull DA, et al. Diuretic strategies in patients with acute decompensated heart failure. N Engl J Med 2011;364(9):797–805.

24. Krum H, Iyngkaran P, Lekawanvijit S. Pharmacologic management of the cardiorenal syndrome in heart failure. Curr Heart Fail Rep 2009;6(2):105–11.

25. Liang KV, Williams AW, Greene EL, et al. Acute decompensated heart failure and the cardiorenal syndrome. Crit Care Med 2008;36(Suppl 1):S75–88.

26. Mills RM, LeJemtel TH, Horton DP, et al. Sustained hemodynamic effects of an infusion of nesiritide (human b-type natriuretic peptide) in heart failure: a randomized, double-blind, placebo-controlled clinical trial. J Am Coll Cardiol 1999;34(1):155–62.

27. Colucci WS, Elkayam U, Horton DP, et al. Intravenous nesiritide, a natriuretic peptide, in the treatment of decompensated congestive heart failure. N Engl J Med 2000;343(4):246–53.

28. Publication Committee for the VMAC Investigators. Intravenous nesiritide vs nitroglycerin for treatment of decompensated congestive heart failure: a randomized controlled trial. JAMA 2002;287(12):1531–40.

29. Butler J, Emerman C, Peacock WF, et al. The efficacy and safety of B-type natriuretic peptide (nesiritide) in patients with renal insufficiency and acutely decompensated congestive heart failure. Nephrol Dial Transplant 2004;19(2):391–9.

30. Sackner-Bernstein JD, Skopicki HA, Aaronson KD. Risk of worsening renal function with nesiritide in patients with acutely decompensated heart failure. Circulation 2005;111(12):1487–91.

31. Sackner-Bernstein JD, Kowalski M, Fox M, et al. Short-term risk of death after treatment with nesiritide for decompensated heart failure: a pooled analysis of randomized controlled trials. JAMA 2005; 293(15):1900–5.

32. Hauptman PJ, Schnitzler MA, Swindle J, et al. Use of nesiritide before and after publications suggesting drug-related risks in patients with acute decompensated heart failure. JAMA 2006;296(15):1877–84.

33. Teerlink JR. Dyspnea as an end point in clinical trials of therapies for acute decompensated heart failure. Am Heart J 2003;145(Suppl 2):S26–33.

34. West RI, Hernandez AF, O'Connor CM, et al. A review of dyspnea in acute heart failure syndromes. Am Heart J 2010;160(2):209–14.

35. Anand IS, Florea VG, Fisher L. Surrogate end points in heart failure. J Am Coll Cardiol 2002; 39(9):1414–21.

36. Stevenson LW, Tillisch JH, Hamilton M, et al. Importance of hemodynamic response to therapy in predicting survival with ejection fraction less than or equal to 20% secondary to ischemic or nonischemic dilated cardiomyopathy. Am J Cardiol 1990;66(19): 1348–54.

37. Lucas C, Johnson W, Hamilton MA, et al. Freedom from congestion predicts good survival despite previous class IV symptoms of heart failure. Am Heart J 2000;140(6):840–7.

38. Packer M, Carver JR, Rodeheffer RJ, et al. Effect of oral milrinone on mortality in severe chronic heart failure. The PROMISE Study Research Group. N Engl J Med 1991;325(21):1468–75.

39. Califf RM, Adams KF, McKenna WJ, et al. A randomized controlled trial of epoprostenol therapy for severe congestive heart failure: the Flolan

International Randomized Survival Trial (FIRST). Am Heart J 1997;134(1):44–54.

40. Cohn JN, Goldstein SO, Greenberg BH, et al. A dose-dependent increase in mortality with vesnarinone among patients with severe heart failure. Vesnarinone Trial Investigators. N Engl J Med 1998; 339(25):1810–6.

41. Binanay C, Califf RM, Hasselblad V, et al. Evaluation study of congestive heart failure and pulmonary artery catheterization effectiveness: the ESCAPE trial. JAMA 2005;294(13):1625–33.

42. Cohn J, Cleland JG, Lubsen J, et al. Unconventional end points in cardiovascular clinical trials: should we be moving away from morbidity and mortality? J Card Fail 2009;15(3):199–205.

43. Gheorghiade M, Konstam MA, Burnett JC Jr, et al. Short-term clinical effects of tolvaptan, an oral vasopressin antagonist, in patients hospitalized for heart failure: the EVEREST Clinical Status Trials. JAMA 2007;297(12):1332–43.

44. Neaton JD, Gray G, Zuckerman BD, et al. Key issues in end point selection for heart failure trials: composite end points. J Card Fail 2005;11(8):567–75.

45. Freemantle N, Calvert M, Wood J, et al. Composite outcomes in randomized trials: greater precision but with greater uncertainty? JAMA 2003;289(19): 2554–9.

46. Fonarow GC, ADHERE Scientific Advisory Committee. The Acute Decompensated Heart Failure National Registry (ADHERE): opportunities to improve care of patients hospitalized with acute decompensated heart failure. Rev Cardiovasc Med 2003;4(Suppl 7):S21–30.

47. Bourge RC, Abraham WT, Adamson PB, et al. Randomized controlled trial of an implantable continuous hemodynamic monitor in patients with advanced heart failure: the COMPASS-HF study. J Am Coll Cardiol 2008;51(11):1073–9.

48. O'Connor CM, Fiuzat M. Is rehospitalization after heart failure admission a marker of poor quality? Time for re-evaluation. J Am Coll Cardiol 2010;56(5):369–71.

49. Givertz MM, Massie BM, Fields TK, et al. The effects of KW-3902, an adenosine A1-receptor antagonist, on diuresis and renal function in patients with acute decompensated heart failure and renal impairment or diuretic resistance. J Am Coll Cardiol 2007; 50(16):1551–60.

50. Gottlieb SS, Brater DC, Thomas I, et al. BG9719 (CVT-124), an A1 adenosine receptor antagonist, protects against the decline in renal function observed with diuretic therapy. Circulation 2002;105(11):1348–53.

51. Weatherley BD, Cotter G, Dittrich HC, et al. Design and rationale of the PROTECT study: a placebo-controlled randomized study of the selective A1 adenosine receptor antagonist rolofylline for patients hospitalized with acute decompensated heart failure and volume overload to assess treatment effect on

congestion and renal function. J Card Fail 2010; 16(1):25–35.

52. Cotter G, Dittrich HC, Weatherley BD, et al. The PROTECT pilot study: a randomized, placebo-controlled, dose-finding study of the adenosine A1 receptor antagonist rolofylline in patients with acute heart failure and renal impairment. J Card Fail 2008; 14(8):631–40.

53. Gottlieb SS, Ticho B, Deykin A, et al. Effects of BG9928, an adenosine A1 receptor antagonist, in patients with congestive heart failure. J Clin Pharmacol 2011;51(6):899–907.

54. Felker GM, Maisel AS. A global rank end point for clinical trials in acute heart failure. Circ Heart Fail 2010;3(5):643–6.

55. Felker GM, Anstrom KJ, Rogers JG. A global ranking approach to end points in trials of mechanical circulatory support devices. J Card Fail 2008;14(5):368–72.

56. Lachin JM. Worst-rank score analysis with informatively missing observations in clinical trials. Control Clin Trials 1999;20(5):408–22.

57. O'Connor CM, Starling RC, Hernandez AF, et al. Effect of nesiritide in patients with acute decompensated heart failure. N Engl J Med 2011;365(1):32–43.

End Point Selection in Acute Decompensated Heart Failure Clinical Trials: Economic End Points

Shelby D. Reed, PhD*, Zubin J. Eapen, MD,
Kevin A. Schulman, MD

KEYWORDS

- Costs and cost analysis • Economics • Medical
- Health care costs • Research design

No health care system is immune from pressures to constrain the rate of growth in health care spending. Outside the United States, most decisions about payment for new technologies are made at the national level with explicit consideration of a fixed budget. Health technology assessment has long been an integral part of decision making for coverage of new drugs and devices in Canada, Australia, the United Kingdom, and many countries throughout Europe.[1] National efforts to consider evidence of cost-effectiveness are spreading to Asia, South America, and Africa.[2,3] In the United States, decision making is decentralized for persons covered by the private insurance market, but largely centralized for patients 65 years or older with traditional fee-for-service Medicare. Although consideration of costs or cost-effectiveness may not be openly endorsed by the private market, adoption of value-based insurance design in which beneficiaries pay higher copayments for lower-value (ie, less cost-effective) therapies is an indication that payers are increasingly scrutinizing coverage decisions. In making coverage decisions for Medicare, the Centers for Medicare & Medicaid Services (CMS) is barred from explicit consideration of cost-effectiveness.

Nevertheless, national coverage determinations have centered on high-cost treatments, and CMS is experimenting with demonstration projects and "coverage with evidence development" and is considering the use of bundled payments that would provide a single payment for all medical services provided during a defined period.[4] For patients admitted with acute decompensated heart failure, this period may include the initial hospitalization plus outpatient services and any readmissions during a 30-day period.

As evidentiary standards for new technologies evolve, economic outcomes are increasingly included as secondary end points in clinical trial protocols to inform decision making. They serve as an important complement to evidence on safety and efficacy and can clarify the value of investing resources in a new drug, device, or program.

For new therapies targeting patients with acute decompensated heart failure (ADHF), the target audience for economic evaluations in the United States depends on whether hospitals will receive an add-on payment in addition to a prospective (ie, fixed) payment for patients admitted with ADHF. If payers do not reimburse beyond the prospective payment rate when a new drug is

The authors have no relevant disclosures. Drs Reed and Schulman have made available online detailed listings of financial disclosures (http://www.dcri.duke.edu/about-us/conflict-of-interest/).
Department of Medicine, Duke Clinical Research Institute, Duke University School of Medicine, PO Box 17969, Durham, NC 27715, USA
* Corresponding author.
E-mail address: shelby.reed@duke.edu

Heart Failure Clin 7 (2011) 529–537
doi:10.1016/j.hfc.2011.06.014
1551-7136/11/$ – see front matter © 2011 Elsevier Inc. All rights reserved.

administered, hospital pharmacy and therapeutics committees must carefully consider the balance of additional costs for the new therapy and its potential impact on inpatient resource use and costs as well as health outcomes for patients. In deciding on whether to provide an add-on payment, payers may consider economic evidence such as the cost-effectiveness of a new drug that can improve patient outcomes and/or reduce downstream costs. Understanding the costs borne by hospitals and payers affects the broad-scale adoption of a new treatment and ultimately its impact on patient outcomes.

COSTS OF ADHF

Spending for heart failure care exemplifies the broader expansion of health care spending. It is the only category of cardiovascular disease for which the prevalence, incidence, hospitalization rate, total burden of mortality, and costs have increased in the past 25 years.[5] ADHF, a constellation of multiple clinical syndromes that result in worsening heart failure requiring hospitalization, is responsible for a considerable portion of the health care costs for persons with heart failure. In the United States alone, more than 1 million hospitalizations annually are attributable to ADHF.[6–10] The total number of hospitalizations is driven by frequent readmission, the rate of which ranges from approximately 9% to 25% at 30 days and 14% to 32% at 90 days, depending on the underlying severity of heart failure and comorbid conditions in the patient population.[11–13]

In 2009, inpatient costs for ADHF totaled $20.1 billion.[14] Not widely recognized, however, is that costs specifically for subsequent heart failure hospitalizations represent only about 15% of total inpatient costs for patients with heart failure.[15] Readmissions for all cardiovascular-related causes (including heart failure) represent about 43% of inpatient costs after an index hospitalization for heart failure. Because patients with heart failure are most frequently hospitalized for other conditions, the impact of a therapy specifically targeting readmission for heart failure is somewhat limited. Whellan and colleagues[15] report that mean inpatient costs to Medicare for heart failure readmissions were $1866 ($2001) in the year after an index hospitalization for heart failure. If an economic evaluation of a new therapy for ADHF is limited to examining costs associated with readmissions for heart failure, the maximum savings that could be expected with a 100% reduction in heart failure readmissions is about $2600 when updating costs to 2010 values[16] (assuming that the trial is targeting patients similar to Medicare

beneficiaries with an initial hospitalization for heart failure). With a 25% reduction, savings ($650) is similar to costs for patented drugs for ADHF (eg, levosimendan, nesiritide). However, it is important to consider that most trial protocols designed to evaluate drugs for ADHF have follow-up periods shorter than 1 year (eg, 30 days, 90 days) and this would expectedly reduce potential savings. Thus, cost savings in the short term may be a difficult goal to achieve. Nevertheless, a drug that adds incrementally to short-term health care costs may prove to be cost-effective if shown to improve patients' quality of life and/or survival. For example, assume that a new therapy costs an additional $500 and reduces inpatient mortality from 12% to 8%. If remaining life expectancy for surviving patients is 4 years, the therapy would be considered cost-effective at approximately $5000 per life-year gained.

INTEGRATING ECONOMIC END POINTS IN CLINICAL TRIALS OF ADHF

Prospectively planned economic evaluations performed alongside clinical trials represent the state of the art in the generation of high-quality evidence on costs, patient outcomes, and cost-effectiveness of new technologies and medical programs to inform coverage decisions. One of the first prospective trial-based economic evaluations was integrated into the Flolan International Randomized Survival Trial (FIRST), a trial evaluating epoprostenol in patients with ADHF, in the early 1990s.[17,18] Since then, economic end points have increasingly been included in study protocols, particularly in phase 3 clinical trials. Growth in the number of trial-based economic evaluations can be attributed to several important advantages.[19] One significant advantage is the acquisition of patient-level data, which allows analysts to apply statistical methods to generate unbiased comparisons of resource use, costs, and effects from the same cohort of patients. Other advantages can include the timeliness of the results to inform decision making at the time of product launch, the ability to evaluate statistical uncertainty associated with the results, and the evaluation of patient subgroups.

Integration of economic end points typically involves additional data elements in the case report form. The amount of data collection required for an economic evaluation depends on the technology or program being evaluated. The selection of economic variables is directed toward resources that represent a significant share of total costs (ie, cost drivers) and those that are expected to differ between treatments. However, collection of resource use should not be limited to that which is believed by the investigator to be disease-related or therapy-related. For example, data on all-cause hospitalizations should be ascertained because a therapy may have unforeseen consequences, either positive or negative, that may result in hospitalization (eg, cyclooxygenase-2 inhibitors). In evaluation of therapies for ADHF, data requirements for economic evaluations largely overlap with those collected for clinical outcomes, including length of stay, use of other medications, and data pertaining to readmissions and emergency department visits. Additional data collection on medical resource use frequently includes outpatient visits to various medical providers (eg, primary care physicians, specialists, nurse practitioners), home visits, and days in skilled nursing or other long-term care facilities. In some cases, data on medical resource use are augmented through collection of hospital bills or other administrative data (eg, medical claims). Incremental data requirements to assign costs to the study intervention are minimal for drugs. For programmatic interventions (eg, case management), information pertaining to supplies, equipment, and personnel time may be collected in the case report form or through a separate survey or time-and-motion study.

Economic protocols in cardiovascular trials frequently include the administration of a preference-based instrument, such as the EQ-5D or Health Utilities Index.[20] Patients' responses to these questionnaires are converted to utility weights—numerical values generally ranging from 0 to 1—which are combined with survival estimates to calculate quality-adjusted life-years. A more comprehensive economic evaluation can include resources that represent patient costs, such as time spent receiving medical care, changes in employment, days missed from work because of poor health, and out-of-pocket expenses. The decision as to whether costs to patients are included in an economic evaluation depends on the study's perspective. A study conducted from the perspective of the health care system would be limited to direct medical costs, whereas a study conducted from the perspective of society or the patient would include costs incurred by patients.

ECONOMIC END POINTS IN RECENT ADHF CLINICAL TRIALS

During the past few years, some trial protocols in ADHF have prospectively integrated economic evaluations, whereas other protocols have not. In the latter cases, analysts have relied on data elements collected for clinical and/or safety end points to conduct retrospective economic evaluations. An overview of economic evaluations for key trials over the recent few years sheds light on the variability in economic end point selection, methods, and results.

UNLOAD Trial

The UNLOAD (Ultrafiltration Versus IV Diuretics for Patients Hospitalized for Acute Decompensated Congestive Heart Failure) trial compared 200 patients hospitalized with ADHF who were randomly assigned to receive ultrafiltration or intravenous diuretics.[13] The primary end points in the trial were weight loss and dyspnea measured at 48 hours. Although a prospectively planned economic evaluation was not integrated into the protocol, several secondary end points in the trial represented counts of resource use including heart failure hospitalizations and unscheduled visits. At 90 days of follow-up, patients randomly assigned to ultrafiltration were less likely to be hospitalized for heart failure (18% vs 32%; $P = .04$) and had fewer readmissions for heart failure (0.22 vs 0.46; $P = .02$), readmission days (1.4 vs 3.8 days; $P = .02$), and unscheduled visits (21% vs 44%; $P = .009$). Using published results from this trial, Bradley and colleagues[21] designed a decision-analysis model to evaluate costs and health outcomes associated with ultrafiltration versus intravenous diuretics.[21] The investigators used Medicare reimbursement rates and estimates of length of stay from CMS to derive an estimated daily inpatient cost for heart failure. They calculated costs associated with ultrafiltration based on the cost of the device, amortized over 5 years, cost for associated service, ultrafiltration filters, nursing time, physician fees, and heparin infusion. They also included probabilities and costs of complications, such as catheter-related bloodstream infections and major bleeding events. The 90-day base-case cost estimates were $13,469 for ultrafiltration and $11,610 for intravenous diuretics.

SURVIVE Trial

De Lissovoy and colleagues[22] performed an economic evaluation of the SURVIVE (Survival of Patients with Acute Heart Failure in Need of Intravenous Inotropic Support) trial, a randomized trial of levosimendan versus dobutamine in 1327 patients with ADHF. At 180 days, mortality (the primary end point) was 26% in the levosimendan group compared with 28% in the dobutamine group ($P = .40$). The investigators conducted the study to inform decision making in Western Europe. Their approach to cost estimation involved multiplying inpatient days by per diem rates from France, Germany, and the United Kingdom. They applied each country's per diem rates to inpatient days for patients enrolled from each country. For patients enrolled in other countries, they applied the average rate from France, Germany, and the United Kingdom.

In the intention-to-treat group and the subgroup that excluded patients with low blood pressure, costs during the index hospitalization were similar in the levosimendan group and the dobutamine group ($P = .94$) when excluding costs for levosimendan. During the 180-day follow-up period, readmissions and inpatient costs were similar between treatment groups in both the intention-to-treat cohort and the subgroup that excluded patients with low blood pressure. They did not report on emergency department visits or outpatient visits.

The reported mean cost for the index hospitalization was an estimated €5060 in the 664 patients randomly assigned to levosimendan and €4952 in the 663 patients randomly assigned to dobutamine. The cost of levosimendan was excluded. Costs during the 180-day follow-up period were reported to be €335 for levosimendan and €323 for dobutamine. Given that the mean numbers of readmissions were 0.73 and 0.86 for the levosimendan and dobutamine groups, respectively, one would expect follow-up costs to be severalfold higher than reported.

Despite the statistically nonsignificant differences in mortality and readmission rates at 180 days, the analysts conducted a cost-effectiveness analysis. The analysts extrapolated survival for patients alive at 180 days by applying a mean estimate of 781 days from the Cooperative North Scandinavian Enalapril Survival Study (CONSENSUS). The analysts concluded that "at an acquisition cost of €600 per vial, there is at least a 50% likelihood that levosimendan is cost effective relative to dobutamine if willingness to pay is equal to or greater than €15,000 per life year gained." This finding includes a great amount of uncertainty in clinical outcomes reflecting a nonsignificant 2 percentage point difference in survival at 180 days.

REVIVE II Trial

De Lissovoy and colleagues[23] performed an economic evaluation of the REVIVE II (second Randomized Multicenter Evaluation of Intravenous Levosimendan Efficacy) study, a randomized trial designed to compare a single 24-hour infusion of levosimendan to placebo, in addition to standard of care, in 600 patients with ADHF. In the intent-to-treat cohort, 90-day mortality was 15.1% in the levosimendan group and 11.6% in the placebo group ($P = .21$). Mortality was higher in the

levosimendan cohort compared with the placebo cohort (26.5% vs 16.3%) among patients with low blood pressure at baseline, whereas mortality was similar in the levosimendan cohort compared with the placebo cohort (8.4% vs 9.1%) among patients with higher blood pressure at baseline. Current labeling for levosimendan cautions that the drug should be used with caution in patients with diastolic blood pressure lower than 60 mm Hg or systolic blood pressure lower than 100 mm Hg. For this reason, the investigators reported 2 sets of results: one for the intention-to-treat cohort and one for the subgroup of patients with higher blood pressure at baseline.

In the intention-to-treat cohort, mean length of stay was 7.0 days in the levosimendan group compared with 9.0 in the placebo group ($P = .008$). Using an externally generated regression model, the analysts assigned inpatient costs on the basis of patient age, sex, days in the intensive care unit, days in the general ward, procedures performed, and whether the patient died during the hospital say. The resulting mean costs for the index hospitalization were approximately $5400 lower in the levosimendan group compared with placebo ($13,590 vs $19,021). However, during the 90-day follow-up period, costs were approximately $2400 higher in the levosimendan group compared with placebo, resulting in a net savings of $3000 at 90 days (90% confidence interval [CI], −$8423 to $2088). In the group with higher blood pressure, patients in the levosimendan group incurred costs that were approximately $2000 lower during the index hospitalization, but they incurred costs that were approximately $1800 higher during the follow-up period, a net savings of approximately $200 that was not statistically significant (90% CI, −$3495 to $3053). If the cost of the drug had been included in the analysis, a net cost increase would have been observed.

A cost-effectiveness study was performed for a non-prespecified subgroup of 388 patients without low blood pressure at baseline. Because of the nonsignificant difference in mortality in this subgroup and variability associated with costs over 90 days, the results included a substantial amount of uncertainty. At a cost of $700 for levosimendan, 68% of simulated results were consistent with cost-effectiveness ratios less than or equal to $50,000 per life-year gained. Almost one-third of the simulations were consistent with decreased survival or cost-effectiveness ratios that surpassed $50,000 per life-year gained. The validity of separate analyses of exploratory subgroups is uncertain especially when the primary analysis is negative.

These completed studies (UNLOAD, SURVIVE, REVIVE II) were retrospective economic evaluations that relied on data collected for evaluating clinical outcomes. However, prospectively planned economic evaluations have recently been incorporated into ADHF trials. A prospective economic evaluation was planned for the PROTECT (A Placebo-controlled Randomized study of rolofylline for patients hospitalized with acute heart failure and volume Overload to assess Treatment Effect on Congestion and renal funcTion) trial, which was designed to compare the safety and efficacy of rolofylline (KW-3902) versus placebo in patients with acute heart failure syndrome, volume overload, and renal impairment.[24] The study objectives for the economic evaluation were to estimate and compare within-trial medical resource use, direct medical costs, and health state utilities between patients treated with rolofylline versus placebo during 60 days of follow-up. The protocol also included a formal cost-effectiveness evaluation to estimate the incremental cost per quality-adjusted life-year for patients treated with rolofylline versus placebo. However, rolofylline was not superior with regard to patient-reported dyspnea, death, or readmission or signs and/symptoms of heart failure relative to placebo.[25]

A prospectively planned economic evaluation was also incorporated into the protocol for ASCEND-HF (Acute Study of Clinical Effectiveness of Nesiritide in Decompensated Heart Failure), a trial designed to evaluate the safety and efficacy of nesiritide in ADHF, with clinical results expected to be presented in late 2010. The economic study objectives are similar to those for PROTECT with the exception that the trial focuses on 30-day end points (instead of 60). In addition, there are likely to be other clinical trial protocols in ADHF with prospectively planned economic evaluations. However, economic end points are rarely reported in publically available sources such as ClinicalTrials.gov. This is unfortunate because of concerns about publication of industry-sponsored trials[26] and potential bias in economic evaluations of industry-sponsored studies.[27,28]

VARIATIONS IN CLINICAL AND ECONOMIC END POINTS ACROSS TRIALS IN ADHF

A lack of success in developing novel therapies for ADHF is partly attributable to the heterogeneity of end points used in clinical trials. No 2 trials conducted in ADHF during the past decade have used the same primary end point.[29] Although economic end points in ADHF clinical trials center on inpatient resource use—particularly length of stay associated with the index hospitalization and readmissions—a great deal of variability exists at a more granular level. The variability stems from variations in the duration of follow-up (eg, 30 days, 60 days,

180 days); the examination of heart failure-related, cardiovascular-related, or all-case hospitalizations; and the inclusion or exclusion of emergency department visits and outpatient resource use.

In addition to variation in the definitions of end points, other types of variations affect their generalizability, including the types of patients enrolled and the geographic distribution of participating sites. In an era of multinational trials, variability in practice patterns is notable for its impact on both clinical and economic end points. Length of stay for the index hospitalization in SURVIVE was approximately twice as long as in REVIVE II (approximately 14 days vs 8 days; see **Table 1**). This result reflected longer stays in countries that participated in SURVIVE, with 26% from France and Germany and 56% from Russia, Poland, and Latvia, compared with the countries participating in REVIVE II (ie, Australia, Israel, and the United States). The shortest stays were reported from UNLOAD, which was limited to sites in the United States. Heart failure is relatively unique in that economic outcomes (ie, hospitalizations) form part of the composite primary clinical end point of many studies. Given this structure, international or regional variability in treatment patterns and access to care can have an unexpected impact on type II statistical error in these studies.

Methodological Issues Inherent to Economic Evaluations

Although published recommendations for conducting trial-based economic evaluations are useful in guiding analysts on major methodological issues,[30] there are numerous choices in terms of study perspective, cost assignment, and analytic methods that can influence the results of economic evaluations and their generalizability. These issues take on greater complexity in the context of multinational clinical trials.[31,32]

As discussed in the introductory paragraph, the target audience for economic evaluations of ADHF therapies will be considered to determine the appropriate perspective for the study. Even within a study, its perspective is critical to its interpretation. In the analysis of the UNLOAD trial by Bradley and colleagues,[21] ultrafiltration had an 86% probability of being more costly than intravenous diuretics from a societal perspective in which the costs of patient inconvenience and urgent care visits were included. This finding was similar to the hospital perspective for which ultrafiltration had a 97% probability of being more costly. However, from a Medicare perspective, in which the analysts incorporated fixed-rate payments for the index hospitalization, readmissions, and unscheduled

Table 1
Recent economic evaluations in acute decompensated heart failure

Trial	Prospective Economic Evaluation?	Follow-up	Inpatient Cost Estimation	Mean Length of Stay for Index Hospitalization	Mean Readmission Days in Follow-up Period
UNLOAD[21]	No	90 d	Per diem rates calculated from Medicare reimbursement and mean length of stay for DRG 127 (heart failure) plus cost for ultrafiltration	Ultrafiltration: 6.3 d; standard care: 5.8 d; $P = .98$	Ultrafiltration: 1.4 d; standard care: 3.8 d; $P = .02$
SURVIVE[22]	No	180 d	Per diem payments for specific diagnoses or procedures in France, Germany, and United Kingdom and mean per diem from these countries for patients in other countries	Levosimendan: 14.3 d; Dobutamine: 14.5 d; $P = .98$	Levosimendan: 11.4 d; Dobutamine: 12.4 d $P = .43$
REVIVE II[23]	No	90 d	Regression model to predict inpatient costs (age, sex, intensive care days, general ward days, procedure, died)	Levosimendan: 7.0 d; standard care: 9.0 d; $P = .008$	Levosimendan: 5.1 d; standard care: 4.4 d; $P = .81$

Abbreviations: REVIVE-II, second Randomized Multicenter Evaluation of Intravenous Levosimendan Efficacy; SURVIVE, Survival of Patients with Acute Heart Failure in Need of Intravenous Inotropic Support; UNLOAD, Ultrafiltration versus IV Diuretics for Patients Hospitalized for Acute Decompensated Congestive Heart Failure.

urgent care visits, ultrafiltration was expected to be cost-saving with greater than 99% probability.

Sources and methods used to assign costs to medical resources documented in the trial case report form will vary across countries and study perspectives. In trials of ADHF, it is important to have an accurate assessment of costs associated with the index hospitalization. In the United States, use of hospital accounting data or hospital bills provides a defensible, objective measure of admission-specific costs (after conversion from charges) for the patients enrolled in the clinical trial. The availability of billing data may be particularly advantageous for ADHF therapies that not only reduce length of stay, but also reduce the intensity of medical care required during the stay. Both the PROTECT and ASCEND-HF protocols included hospital bill collection for US sites.

Outside the United States, however, hospital bills are rarely available. Therefore, additional or alternative costing strategies are typically required. One alternative strategy is the use of a regression model that predicts costs based on resource use measures, such as hospital days in various wards, procedures, patient characteristics, and clinical outcomes, such as the model applied in REVIVE II.[24] Another inpatient costing strategy is the assignment of per diem costs (ie, cost per day) to days in the hospital or days in specific wards. Per diem costing is sensitive to differences in length of stay between treatments but is not sensitive to differences in intensity of care across stays of the same duration. A simpler method is to assign a single fixed cost to represent the total cost of a hospital stay regardless of differences in length of stay. The latter method may be preferable in multinational studies in which there are wide variations in length of stay across countries participating in the trial to avoid misestimated costs when applying one country's per diem rate to hospital stays for patients in other countries where the length of stay may be substantially different from in the country of interest.

There are 2 important issues to note with regard to the per diem and fixed cost methods. The first is that both methods underestimate the true variation in inpatient costs across hospital stays (even of the same duration). As a result, statistical variation is underestimated and comparisons are more likely to (falsely) demonstrate statistical significance.

The second issue applies to the per diem costing approach. Because the most resource-intensive hospital days typically occur upon admission, applying the same per diem to all hospital days in an economic evaluation will tend to overestimate cost savings resulting from shorter hospital stays.[33]

The issues discussed previously pertain to sources of variation in economic evaluations resulting from different methodological choices. A separate issue is that results from analyses of clinical and economic end points for a single trial may appear to be discrepant. Analyses of readmission as a clinical end point typically focus on the time to the first readmission, whereas economic analyses focus on the total number of admissions. In HF-ACTION (Heart Failure: A Controlled Trial Investigating Outcomes of Exercise Training), after adjusting for prognostic variables, an 11% reduction was reported for all-cause mortality or hospitalization based on a time-to-event analysis. However, analyses of the cumulative number of events revealed similar numbers of hospitalizations in each treatment group (2297 vs 2332; $P = .92$) and similar numbers of deaths (189 vs 198; $P = .70$). Also, short-term benefits reported for clinical outcomes may not translate into improved economic outcomes. For example, improvements in a short-term benefit like dyspnea do not necessarily correlate with changes in preference-based measures of quality of life (ie, health utilities) or short-term or long-term measures of resource use. Without an established relationship between short-term improvements and longer-term changes in quality of life, resource use, or survival, economic modeling is not defensible.

Next Steps

An international working group recently called for better design of clinical trials in ADHF, particularly with regard to standardization. Greater consensus is needed on both clinical and economic end points. As standardization evolves for the assessment of clinical outcomes, standardization of economic end points will likely follow. Consistent use of the same period of follow-up would help immensely. Also, repeated use of the same short-term measures may allow researchers to establish whether there are consistent and reliable associations between short-term and long-term outcomes. Finally, efforts to reduce variability related to practice pattern variation may increase the signal-to-noise ratio for assessment of ADHF therapies in clinical trials.

Novel therapies in ADHF face the difficult challenge of proving an incremental benefit over existing strategies, most of which consists of low-cost drugs such as furosemide and dobutamine. These lower-cost drugs may be used successfully to treat many patients. New therapies will provide the greatest economic value if they are targeted to patients who do not adequately respond to older therapies and patients who are predicted to incur higher costs. A great deal of interest is focused on targeting treatments toward high-risk patients and those who are most likely to benefit through integration of biomarkers such as b-type natriuretic peptide (BNP) or N-terminal proBNP (NT-proBNP). In the design phase of a clinical trial, having some knowledge about the expected costs of a new therapy would be useful in determining whether the therapy could prove to be cost effective in lower-risk and higher-risk patient populations. With this information, it may be advantageous to more narrowly define a study population to patients likely to have higher rates of downstream resource use.

SUMMARY

Evidence from formal cost-effectiveness analyses will increasingly be used by third-party payers and national health systems to steer expenditures toward higher-value, although not necessarily inexpensive, treatments. However, without additional payments to hospitals for new ADHF treatments, decision making at the hospital level is largely informed with reliable information on inpatient costs and cost offsets in a shorter time frame. Thus, plans for economic evaluations of new ADHF therapies should include within-trial comparisons of resource use and costs, as well as principled plans to conduct formal cost-effectiveness analyses.

In conclusion, the selection of economic end points in ADHF clinical trials requires prospectively planned evaluations that are developed in tandem with clinical end points. Integrating economic end points with concrete postdischarge clinical outcomes will provide meaningful descriptions of the resources needed to provide beneficial treatment for patients and an accurate assessment of the treatment's incremental value in the setting of ADHF.

REFERENCES

1. Clement FM, Harris A, Li JJ, et al. Using effectiveness and cost-effectiveness to make drug coverage decisions: a comparison of Britain, Australia, and Canada. JAMA 2009;302:1437–43.
2. Kristensen FB, Mäkelä M, Neikter SA, et al. European network for health technology assessment,

EUnetHTA: planning, development, and implementation of a sustainable European network for health technology assessment. Int J Technol Assess Health Care 2009;25(Suppl 2):107–16.

3. Oortwijn W, Mathijssen J, Banta D. The role of health technology assessment on pharmaceutical reimbursement in selected middle-income countries. Health Policy 2010;95:174–84.

4. Hackbarth G, Reischauer R, Mutti A. Collective accountability for medical care—toward bundled Medicare payments. N Engl J Med 2008;359:3–5.

5. Hunt SA, American College of Cardiology; American Heart Association Task Force on Practice Guidelines (Writing Committee to Update the 2001 Guidelines for the Evaluation and Management of Heart Failure). ACC/AHA 2005 guideline update for the diagnosis and management of chronic heart failure in the adult: a report of the American College of Cardiology/American Heart Association Task Force on Practice Guidelines (Writing Committee to Update the 2001 Guidelines for the Evaluation and Management of Heart Failure). J Am Coll Cardiol 2005;46:e1–82.

6. Dickstein K, Cohen-Solal A, Filippatos G, et al, Task Force for Diagnosis and Treatment of Acute and Chronic Heart Failure 2008 of European Society of Cardiology. ESC Guidelines for the diagnosis and treatment of acute and chronic heart failure 2008: the Task Force for the Diagnosis and Treatment of Acute and Chronic Heart Failure 2008 of the European Society of Cardiology. Developed in collaboration with the Heart Failure Association of the ESC (HFA) and endorsed by the European Society of Intensive Care Medicine (ESICM). Eur Heart J 2008;29:2388–442.

7. Fang J, Mensah GA, Croft JB, et al. Heart failure-related hospitalization in the US, 1979 to 2004. J Am Coll Cardiol 2008;52:428–34.

8. Rosamond W, Flegal K, Furie K, et al. Heart disease and stroke statistics—2008 update: a report from the American Heart Association Statistics Committee and Stroke Statistics Subcommittee. Circulation 2008;117:e25–146.

9. Nieminen MS, Brutsaert D, Dickstein K, et al. Euro-Heart Failure Survey II (EHFS II): a survey on hospitalized acute heart failure patients: description of population. Eur Heart J 2006;27:2725–36.

10. Jessup M, Abraham WT, Casey DE, et al. 2009 focused update: ACCF/AHA Guidelines for the Diagnosis and Management of Heart Failure in Adults: a report of the American College of Cardiology Foundation/American Heart Association Task Force on Practice Guidelines: developed in collaboration with the International Society for Heart and Lung Transplantation. Circulation 2009;119:1977–2016.

11. Ko DT, Tu JV, Masoudi FA, et al. Quality of care and outcomes of older patients with heart failure hospitalized in the United States and Canada. Arch Intern Med 2005;165:2486–92.

12. Ross HS, Chen J, Lin Z, et al. Recent national trends in readmission rates after heart failure hospitalization. Circ Heart Fail 2010;3:97–103.

13. Costanzo MR, Guglin ME, Saltzberg MT, et al. Ultrafiltration versus intravenous diuretics for patients hospitalized for acute decompensated heart failure. J Am Coll Cardiol 2007;49:675–83.

14. Lloyd-Jones D, Adams R, Carnethon M, et al. Heart disease and stroke statistics—2009 update: a report from the American Heart Association Statistics Committee and Stroke Statistics Subcommittee. Circulation 2009;119(3):e21–181.

15. Whellan DJ, Greiner MA, Schulman KA, et al. Costs of inpatient care among Medicare beneficiaries with heart failure, 2001 to 2004. Circ Cardiovasc Qual Outcomes 2010;3:33–40.

16. US Department of Labor, Bureau of Labor Statistics. Consumer Price Index-All Urban Consumers. US Medical Care. Available at: http://data.bls.gov/cgi-bin/surveymost?cu. Accessed August 18, 2010.

17. Schulman KA, Glick H, Buxton M, et al. The economic evaluation of the FIRST study: design of a prospective analysis alongside a multinational phase III clinical trial. Flolan International Randomized Survival Trial. Control Clin Trials 1996;17:304–15.

18. Schulman KA, Buxton M, Glick H, et al. Results of the economic evaluation of the FIRST study. A multinational prospective economic evaluation. FIRST Investigators. Flolan International Randomized Survival Trial. Int J Technol Assess Health Care 1996;12:698–713.

19. Gray AM. Cost-effectiveness analyses alongside randomised clinical trials. Clin Trials 2006;3:538–42.

20. Dyer MT, Goldsmith KA, Sharples LS, et al. A review of health utilities using the EQ-5D in studies of cardiovascular disease. Health Qual Life Outcomes 2010;8:13.

21. Bradley SM, Levy WC, Veenstra DL. Cost-consequences of ultrafiltration for acute heart failure: a decision model analysis. Circ Cardiovasc Qual Outcomes 2009;2:566–73.

22. de Lissovoy G, Fraeman K, Salon J, et al. The costs of treating acute heart failure: an economic analysis of the SURVIVE trial. J Med Econ 2008;11:415–29.

23. de Lissovoy G, Fraeman K, Teerlink JR, et al. Hospital costs for treatment of acute heart failure: economic analysis of the REVIVE II study. Eur J Health Econ 2010;11:185–93.

24. Weatherley BD, Cotter G, Dittrich HC, et al. Design and rationale of the PROTECT study: a placebo-controlled randomized study of the selective A1 adenosine receptor antagonist rolofylline for patients hospitalized with acute decompensated heart failure and volume overload to assess treatment effect on

congestion and renal function. J Card Fail 2010;16:25–35.

25. Cleland JG, Coletta AP, Yassin A, et al. Clinical trials update from the European Society of Cardiology Meeting 2009: AAA, RELY, PROTECT, ACTIVE-I, European CRT survey, German pre-SCD II registry, and MADIT-CRT. Eur J Heart Fail 2009;11:1214–9.

26. Bourgeois FT, Murthy S, Mandl KD. Outcome reporting among drug trials registered in ClinicalTrials.gov. Ann Intern Med 2010;153:158–66.

27. Bell CM, Urbach DR, Ray JG, et al. Bias in published cost effectiveness studies: systematic review. BMJ 2006;332:699–703.

28. Neumann PJ, Fang CH, Cohen JT. 30 years of pharmaceutical cost-utility analyses: growth, diversity and methodological improvement. Pharmacoeconomics 2009;27:861–72.

29. Felker GM, Pang PS, Adams KF, et al. Clinical trials of pharmacological therapies in acute heart failure

syndromes: lessons learned and directions forward. Circ Heart Fail 2010;3:314–25.

30. Ramsey S, Willke R, Briggs A, et al. Best practices for cost-effectiveness analysis alongside clinical trials: an ISPOR RCT-CEA Task Force report. Value Health 2005;8:521–33.

31. Reed SD, Anstrom KJ, Bakhai A, et al. Conducting economic evaluations alongside multinational clinical trials: toward a research consensus. Am Heart J 2005;149:434–43.

32. Sculpher MJ, Pang FS, Manca A, et al. Generalisability in economic evaluation studies in healthcare: a review and case studies. Health Technol Assess 2004;8:1–192.

33. Reed SD, Friedman JY, Gnanasakthy A, et al. Comparison of hospital costing methods in an economic evaluation of a multinational clinical trial. Int J Technol Assess Health Care 2003;19:396–406.

Conduct of Clinical Trials in Acute Heart Failure: Regional Differences in Heart Failure Clinical Trials

Mona Fiuzat, PharmD[a],*, Robert M. Califf, MD[a,b]

KEYWORDS

• Heart failure • Regional differences • Clinical trials

Clinical trials are often conducted globally. A recent study found that approximately one-third of phase 3 industry-sponsored trials (157 of 509) in the ClinicalTrials.gov registry were being conducted solely outside the United States.[1] Differences in standard of care, patient populations including genetic and phenotypic differences, disease etiologies, rates of comorbidities, ascertainment of endpoints, and differences in concomitant therapies and medical culture may influence subsequent outcomes. Because many cardiovascular trials have demonstrated differences in clinical outcomes by continent and geographic region, careful consideration of these factors is warranted.[2–6] Heart failure trials have also demonstrated varying results based on geographic region of the world.[7–9]

Despite these reports, little consensus has emerged regarding how these results should be evaluated. This article reviews the differences in cardiovascular trial results by geographic region, offers potential explanations for these differences, and suggests methods for standardization of trial results.

RATIONALE FOR MULTIREGIONAL CLINICAL TRIALS

The goal of late-phase heart failure clinical trials is to define the balance of risk and benefit for the use of a strategy, drug, or device. The need for multiregional clinical trials stems both from valid scientific concerns about variability in outcomes and treatment response, and because of logistic pressure to meet compressed timelines.

Scientifically, it is possible that the balance of risk and benefit may be affected by the genetic makeup of the individual, but it may be even more affected by the medical culture in which health care is delivered or the local culture with regard to adherence and use of alternative therapies. Thus, it is understandable that most countries would prefer to have representation in clinical trials before a new therapy is allowed to be marketed. For example, the response to anticoagulation varies in different regions, partly because of differences in diet and partly because of differences in the distributions of polymorphisms controlling drug metabolism variation. Similarly, one would expect a different response to add-on therapy in a population optimally treated for heart failure compared with a population with little additional background therapy. A factor now being recognized as important is the excess rate of nonadherence, dropout, and lost to follow-up rates in the United States compared with most other countries. Obviously, all of these factors bias toward a smaller treatment effect, since a treatment effect cannot occur if the research participant does not take the assigned treatment.

Additionally, large sample sizes are required to detect the kind of modest differences seen with most therapies. To meet reasonable timelines,

---

[a] Duke University Medical Center, 2400 Pratt Street, Room 8011, Durham, NC 27710, USA
[b] Duke Translational Medicine Institute, Durham, NC, USA
* Corresponding author.
E-mail address: mona.fiuzat@duke.edu

Heart Failure Clin 7 (2011) 539–544
doi:10.1016/j.hfc.2011.06.004
1551-7136/11/$ – see front matter © 2011 Elsevier Inc. All rights reserved.

larger trials involving multiple regions have become the norm.

REVIEW OF CLINICAL TRIALS IN HEART FAILURE

The US Food and Drug Administration (FDA) has recently evaluated a series of cardiovascular outcome trials with regard to the size of the treatment effect within the United States compared with the rest of world. A highly significant difference was found, with a much smaller treatment effect within the United States versus rest of world. The analysis does not provide insight about the reason for this difference.

One of the first evaluations of this issue in heart failure was the Flolan International Randomized Survival Trial (FIRST) of epoprostenol versus placebo, in which 471 patients with New York Heart Association (NYHA) class 3b/4 heart failure were enrolled in North America and Europe.[7] The trial was terminated early due to a trend toward harm in patients treated with epoprostenol. In a subgroup analysis, patients enrolled from outside North America showed a greater trend toward detriment when treated with epoprostenol (**Fig. 1**), and patients in North America had a higher overall mortality. Investigators at the time speculated this may have been due to higher use of dobutamine, or higher doses of digoxin used in US patients,

thus increasing mortality but producing a better chance of benefit from epoprostenol. Further, management of chronic indwelling catheters may have been more common at the time in the United States, thereby reducing rates of sepsis complications or death.

Recent analyses from the Efficacy of Vasopressin Antagonism in Heart Failure: Outcome Study with Tolvaptan (EVEREST) demonstrated similar regional differences in outcomes.[8] In 4133 patients with worsening heart failure receiving either tolvaptan or placebo, the unadjusted 1-year mortality was highest among North American patients (n = 1251) at 30.4% (confidence interval [CI] 27.6–33.1), while the mortality in patients in South America (n = 699), Western Europe (n = 564), and Eastern Europe (n = 1619) was 27.2% (CI 23.3–30.8), 27.1% (CI 23.0–31.1), and 20.5% (CI 18.1–22.8), respectively (**Fig. 2**).

In chronic heart failure, the same international differences in treatment response have been noted. In particular, beta-blockers have been the cornerstone of therapy in treating heart failure patients worldwide; however, O'Connor and colleagues[9] recently presented the results of a systematic overview analysis demonstrating the differences between United States versus the worldwide cohorts in large beta-blocker trials in heart failure. In this study, the landmark β-blocker survival trials were compared: the Metoprolol

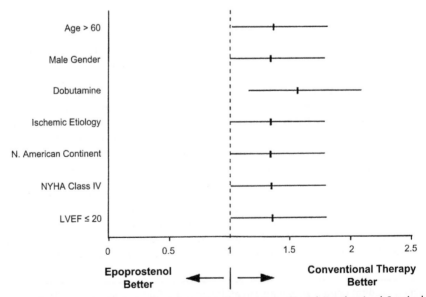

Odds of treatment effect after adjusting for the following factors:

Fig. 1. Regional influence on treatment effect from the Flolan International Randomized Survival Trial (FIRST) trial. Odds ratios and confidence intervals for effects of epoprostenol on mortality rates as function of key baseline characteristics. LVEF, left ventricular ejection fraction; NYHA, New York Heart Association. (*From* Califf RM, Adams KF, McKenna WJ, et al. A randomized controlled trial of epoprostenol therapy for severe congestive heart failure: the Flolan International Randomized Survival Trial (FIRST). Am Heart J 1997;134:51; with permission.)

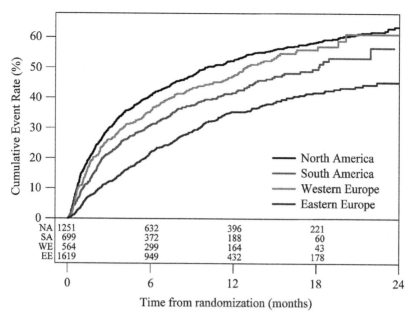

Fig. 2. Cumulative mortality by region from the EVEREST (Efficacy of Vasopressin Antagonism in Heart Failure: Outcome Study with Tolvaptan) trial. (*From* Blair JE, Zannad F, Konstam MA, et al. Continental differences in clinical characteristics, management, and outcomes in patients hospitalized with worsening heart failure results from the EVEREST (Efficacy of Vasopressin Antagonism in Heart Failure: Outcome Study with Tolvaptan) program. J Am Coll Cardiol 2008;52:1644; with permission.)

Controlled-Release Randomized Intervention Trial in Heart Failure (MERIT-HF), The Cardiac Insufficiency Bisoprolol Study (CIBIS-II), the Carvedilol Prospective Randomized Cumulative Survival Trial (COPERNICUS), and the Beta-blocker Evaluation of Survival Trial (BEST).[10–13] In MERIT-HF, metoprolol reduced mortality by 34% compared with placebo; a significant mortality risk reduction of 34% was also seen with bisprolol in CIBIS-II, and a 35% reduction was with carvedilol in COPERNICUS. In contrast, BEST showed a nonsignificant 13% risk reduction in mortality in patients treated with bucindolol versus placebo. Most patients recruited into MERIT-HF, CIBIS-II, and COPERNICUS were white European patients (73%, 100%, and 79%, respectively), while BEST recruited only patients in the United States and Canada (97.7% and 2.3%, respectively). In this analysis, when the US cohorts alone were evaluated, the magnitude of β-blocker survival effect was either diminished compared with the effect in all other countries (hazard ratio [HR] 0.80) or neutral (HR 1.05) in US populations included in COPERNICUS (n = 482) and MERIT-HF (n = 1071), respectively. These results are comparable to the magnitude of β-blocker survival effect (HR 0.87) observed in the US patient population in BEST.

POTENTIAL EXPLANATIONS FOR FINDINGS

These findings may be explained by a number of factors, including differences in the populations studied as well as different practice patterns across geographic regions.

In EVEREST, there were substantial differences in heart failure severity, etiology, and management. When examining the population differences in the regions from EVEREST, the North American population was older and had a higher number of black patients and higher average weight (kg) compared with the other regions. Similar differences have been noted in other trials and registries in North American patients compared with a European population.[14–17] In EVEREST as well as other trials, the approach to revascularization and device use has been very different. Revascularization procedures, pacemaker use, and implantable cardioverter-defibrillator (ICD) use tend to be more common in a North American population. In-hospital mortality and length of hospital stay have also demonstrated significant variability between the United States and Europe.[14–18]

There are clear differences in baseline characteristics in the populations studied in the large β-blocker trials. Domanski and colleagues[19] conducted a comparative analysis that altered the entry criteria for the BEST study population to achieve conformity with those from CIBIS-II, MERIT-HF, and COPERNICUS. This resulted in exclusion of patients with systolic blood pressure less than 100 mm Hg, heart rate less than 60 beats per minute, and age older than 80 years (exclusion criteria employed in those trials). The BEST comparison subgroup was modified to more closely reflect the racial demographics reported for patients enrolled in CIBIS-II and MERIT-HF. Patients were generally comparable with respect to age, race, sex, NYHA functional class, systolic blood pressure, heart rate, and left ventricular ejection fraction (LVEF). Results of this analysis showed a slight reduction in the annual death rate in placebo-treated patients in BEST, and a reduction in the calculated HR for mortality to 0.77 (95% CI 0.65–0.92). When this comparison was used, there was a statistically significant improvement in survival for bucindolol compared with placebo patients ($P = .0041$). This comparative analysis suggested that based on annualized placebo survival, individuals enrolled in BEST and COPERNICUS were at higher risk for death than those enrolled in either MERIT-HF or CIBIS-II; thus, the relative comparisons of the treatment benefit of these studies is complicated by the differing baseline severity of disease. In addition, recent publications from the DNA substudy in BEST have documented variations in genetic polymorphisms that have shown differential response to the beta-blocker bucindolol.[20–22] Variations in allele frequencies among different populations and ethnic groups may likely play a role in the differential response to therapies.

POTENTIAL METHODS FOR STANDARDIZATION

Despite these differences in treatment benefit observed by region in clinical trials, it is likely that the trial results are generalizable to a global population. This may become apparent when populations are compared using a standardized cohort based on baseline characteristics, as well as post-randomization treatments, including the use of evidence-based medicines, device implementation, rates of revascularization, and disease management strategies.

In the case of beta-blockers, there is a clear demonstration of mortality benefit in heart failure patients. A well-defined understanding of the mechanism of treatment benefit has established a therapeutic rationale for the use of these drugs, and they are a cornerstone of therapy for survival and prevention of hospitalization in these patients.

How would such standardization for comparisons occur? This is a critical question as trials continue to be conducted globally. It is important for regulatory agencies to support the standardization and applicability of research in the determination of safety and efficacy of proposed treatments.

Overall Trial Sample Size

In future trials, there should be an attempt to obtain large sample sizes within US and non-US cohorts, and prespecify analysis based on region. Trials should have enough events to estimate the overall treatment effect and rule out regional effect with reasonable power. Importantly, baseline and treatment characteristics, as well as postrandomization treatments, should be captured so that these can be examined in an adjusted analysis. Additionally, this would allow the possibility of stratifying based on geographic location and baseline risk factors.

Differences in Biology

As the field is progressing in identifying genetic factors that may influence disease progression, risk stratification, and treatment response, it may be crucial to collect genetic information routinely in clinical trials. While this field is still evolving, data have shown differential response to treatments based on genetic polymorphisms, although the data have not been conclusive.[20,21,23–26] Perhaps the differences seen in clinical trials are not explained by geographic region, but more likely by the biologic variations of regional populations. Trials should include the early collection of genetic, metabolic, and biomarker information. This information may then be tested by region, to detect differences in biologic effects.

Differences in Enrollment Criteria

When conducting clinical trials globally, enrollment criteria must be general enough to allow broad participation such that demographics reflect a true population, however, with some specificity to ensure enrollment of true disease patients. One such tool to assist in this challenge is the use of biomarkers. Standardization of simple methods to ensure a true acute heart failure population could include brain natriuretic peptides (BNP) or N-terminal BNP (NT-proBNP) measurements, as well as left ventricular ejection fraction (LVEF) cut-offs. Novel biomarkers specific to heart failure are also being investigated, which may provide useful additional tools in future trials.

Differences in Standards of Care

There are large variations in standards of care, as well as inconsistency in the use of clinical practice guidelines. Concomitant therapies should be followed closely, as well as the use of devices such as ICDs and pacemakers. Regional differences may be minimized by excluding certain therapies, such as inotropes, or by requiring standardized therapies (such as intravenous diuretics as inclusion criteria). Further, treatment-naïve patients should not be used as a measure of efficacy that is generalized to well-treated patients.

Different Cultural Practices

A key challenge critical to acute heart failure studies is length of stay (LOS). Readmission rates are inversely proportional to the initial LOS, and this has been shown to be clearly different in the United States versus other regions of the world. In the Italian Heart Survey and European Heart Failure Survey, average lengths of stay were 9 and 11 days, respectively, as compared with the US ADHERE and OPTIMIZE registries, where average length of stay was 4 days.[14–18] It may be necessary to alter endpoints based on this phenomenon. Perhaps a different measurement should be used when studies are conducted globally, or countries with similar rehospitalization rates or LOS should be included. Similarly, it may be necessary to standardize based on rates of device use (ICD, pacemakers, left ventricular assist device) in various regions.

Random Variation

Sophisticated analyses are needed to minimize this challenge. Other useful aids may include enrollment quotas for various regions of the world. While this may increase the timeline and costs associated with clinical trials, it may be an important factor when identifying safety and efficacy across a spectrum of patients.

Other suggested strategies may include rigorous training of investigators in the design, conduct, and ethical oversight of trials, which would allow researchers to engage more fully in multinational clinical research with a standardized approach.

While numerous heart failure trials have enrolled patients internationally, few have reported results by geographic region of enrollment. Recently, the results of the largest acute heart failure registry, Acute Study of Clinical Effectiveness of Nesiritide in Decompensated Heart Failure, were revealed. This trial enrolled over 7000 patients internationally, with nearly half of the patients enrolled from North America. The results by geographic region are highly anticipated and were prespecified.[27]

Clearly, long-term solutions to standardize the globalization of clinical research are needed. Support from industry, academia, and regulatory agencies will help to reach consensus on these issues. Results from internationally conducted clinical trials should be interpreted with attention to response by geographic region, and generalizability of results across these populations.

REFERENCES

1. Glickman SW, McHutchison JG, Peterson ED, et al. Ethical and scientific implications of the globalization of clinical research. N Engl J Med 2009;360: 816–23.
2. Orlandini A, Diaz R, Wojdyla D, et al. Outcomes of patients in clinical trials with ST-segment elevation myocardial infarction among countries with different gross national incomes. Eur Heart J 2006;27: 527–33.
3. Black HR, Elliott WJ, Grandits G, et al. Results of the Controlled ONset Verapamil INvestigation of Cardiovascular Endpoints (CONVINCE) trial by geographical region. J Hypertens 2005;23:1099–106.
4. The PURSUIT Trial Investigators. Inhibition of platelet glycoprotein IIb/IIIa with eptifibatide in patients with acute coronary syndromes. Platelet Glycoprotein IIb/IIIa in Unstable Angina: receptor suppression using integrilin therapy. N Engl J Med 1998;339:436–43.
5. Yusuf S, Hawken S, Ounpuu S, et al. Effect of potentially modifiable risk factors associated with myocardial infarction in 52 countries (the INTERHEART study): case–control study. Lancet 2004;364:937–52.
6. Van de Werf F, Topol EJ, Lee KL, et al. Variations in patient management and outcomes for acute myocardial infarction in the United States and other countries. Results from the GUSTO trial. Global Utilization of Streptokinase and Tissue Plasminogen Activator for Occluded Coronary Arteries. JAMA 1995;273:1586–91.
7. Califf RM, Adams KF, McKenna WJ, et al. A randomized controlled trial of epoprostenol therapy for severe congestive heart failure: the Flolan International Randomized Survival Trial (FIRST). Am Heart J 1997;134:44–54.
8. Blair JE, Zannad F, Konstam MA, et al. Continental differences in clinical characteristics, management, and outcomes in patients hospitalized with worsening heart failure results from the EVEREST (Efficacy of Vasopressin Antagonism in Heart Failure: outcome Study with Tolvaptan) program. J Am Coll Cardiol 2008;52:1640–8.
9. O'Connor C, Koch B, Fiuzat MK, et al. All-cause mortality endpoint comparison in large beta-blocker heart failure trials: United States (US) vs

Rest of World (ROW) [abstract]. J Am Coll Cardiol 2009;53(Suppl):A154.

10. The CIBIS-II Investigators. The Cardiac Insufficiency Bisoprolol Study II (CIBIS-II): a randomised trial. Lancet 1999;353:9–13.

11. The MERIT-HF Study Investigators. Effect of metoprolol CR/XL in chronic heart failure: metoprolol CR/XL randomised intervention trial in congestive heart failure (MERIT-HF). Lancet 1999;353:2001–7.

12. Packer M, Fowler MB, Roecker EB, et al. Effect of carvedilol on the morbidity of patients with severe chronic heart failure: results of the carvedilol prospective randomized cumulative survival (COPERNICUS) study. Circulation 2002;106:2194–9.

13. Beta-blocker evaluation of survival trial investigators. A trial of the beta-blocker bucindolol in patients with advanced chronic heart failure. N Engl J Med 2001; 344:1659–67.

14. Cleland JG, Swedberg K, Follath F, et al. The Euro-Heart Failure survey programme—a survey on the quality of care among patients with heart failure in Europe. Part 1: patient characteristics and diagnosis. Eur Heart J 2003;24:442–63.

15. Komajda M, Follath F, Swedberg K, et al. The Euro-Heart Failure Survey programme—a survey on the quality of care among patients with heart failure in Europe. Part 2: treatment. Eur Heart J 2003;24:464–74.

16. Fonarow GC, Abraham WT, Albert NM, et al. Prospective evaluation of beta-blocker use at the time of hospital discharge as a heart failure performance measure: results from OPTIMIZE-HF. J Card Fail 2007;13:722–31.

17. Abraham WT, Adams KF, Fonarow GC, et al. In-hospital mortality in patients with acute decompensated heart failure requiring intravenous vasoactive medications: an analysis from the Acute Decompensated Heart Failure National Registry (ADHERE). J Am Coll Cardiol 2005;46:57–64.

18. Tavazzi L, Maggioni AP, Lucci D, et al. Nationwide survey on acute heart failure in cardiology ward services in Italy. Eur Heart J 2006;27:1207–15.

19. Domanski MJ, Krause-Steinrauf H, Massie BM, et al. A comparative analysis of the results from 4 trials of beta-blocker therapy for heart failure: BEST, CIBIS-II, MERIT-HF, and COPERNICUS. J Card Fail 2003; 9:354–63.

20. Liggett SB, Mialet-Perez J, Thaneemit-Chen S, et al. A polymorphism within a conserved beta(1)-adrenergic receptor motif alters cardiac function and beta-blocker response in human heart failure. Proc Natl Acad Sci U S A 2006;103:11288–93.

21. Bristow MR, Murphy GA, Krause-Steinrauf H, et al. An {alpha}2C-Adrenergic receptor polymorphism alters the norepinephrine lowering effects and therapeutic response of the beta blocker bucindolol in chronic heart failure. Circ Heart Fail 2010;3(1):21–8.

22. O'Connor CM, Fiuzat MC, Anand I, et al. Additive effects of b1389 Arg/Gly and a2c 322–325 Wt/Del Adrenergic Receptor Genotype Combinations on Morbidity and Mortality in the BEST Trial [abstract]. J Card Fail 2008;14(Suppl 1):S69.

23. de Groote P, Helbecque N, Lamblin N, et al. Association between beta-1 and beta-2 adrenergic receptor gene polymorphisms and the response to beta-blockade in patients with stable congestive heart failure. Pharmacogenet Genomics 2005;15:137–42.

24. Mialet Perez J, Rathz DA, Petrashevskaya NN, et al. Beta 1-adrenergic receptor polymorphisms confer differential function and predisposition to heart failure. Nat Med 2003;9:1300–5.

25. Mason DA, Moore JD, Green SA, et al. A gain-of-function polymorphism in a G-protein coupling domain of the human beta1-adrenergic receptor. J Biol Chem 1999;274:12670–4.

26. McNamara DM, Holubkov R, Janosko K, et al. Pharmacogenetic interactions between beta-blocker therapy and the angiotensin-converting enzyme deletion polymorphism in patients with congestive heart failure. Circulation 2001;103:1644–8.

27. O'Connor CM, Starling RC, Hernandez AF, et al. Effect of nesiritide in patients with acute decompensated heart failure. N Engl J Med 2011;365:32–43.

Site-Based Research in Acute Heart Failure

Patricia A. Adams, BSN, RN

KEYWORDS

- Acute heart failure • Clinical trials • Site-based research

The conduct of clinical trials in acute heart failure has arrived at a critical point. The authors of the recently published "Heart Failure Society of America 2010 Comprehensive Heart Failure Guidelines" describe a "paucity of controlled clinical trial data"[1] with which to write guidelines for the treatment of acute heart failure. At the same time, the systems used to conduct clinical trials have been described as inefficient, lacking infrastructure, and enormously expensive.[2,3]

Much has been written regarding the conduct of clinical trials at a site. Examples include the principal investigator (PI) responsibilities, ethics, good clinical practice guidelines, regulatory compliance, equipoise, subject recruitment and retention, and human subject protection. However, very few publications discuss the organization of the clinical research site, which is the operational unit responsible for the conduct of clinical research in the patient care setting. The site has been described as the "fundamental unit of clinical research" and also as being "largely underappreciated in the clinical research enterprise."[4] Traditionally organized around a single investigator, the site structure has typically been assembled for a single project and then disassembled at the conclusion of the project. This repetitive reorganization can lead to inefficiencies in staffing, training, experience retention, and expense.

An alternate model is the development of a site-based research (SBR) unit, an operating business unit responsible for conducting a portfolio of research projects in a therapeutic area. The SBR is responsible for the financial accountability, regulatory compliance, and academic productivity.

DESIGNING THE SBR FOR ACUTE HEART FAILURE
Engaging the Team Members and Key Personnel

The key personnel of the heart failure SBR are the heart failure faculty, medical director, lead coordinator, clinical research coordinators (CRCs), and clinical trial assistants. The heart failure faculty evaluates potential research protocols for feasibility and scientific merit. The medical director is responsible for the process of choosing projects, conducting scientifically important research, and complying with SBR operation and finance policies. The lead coordinator is responsible for hiring, training, deployment, and guidance of the coordinating staff conducting trials in both inpatient and outpatient settings. The heart failure SBR is supported by a central infrastructure that includes human resources, a financial manager, and a research manager.

The heart failure research key personnel will need to collaborate with the emergency department (ED) personnel. Patients with acute heart failure may be admitted directly from home or the outpatient clinics. Primarily they present to the ED[5] and spend several hours in that location.[5] There is a need for collaboration with ED physicians, ED research coordinators, and ED nursing staff to recruit subjects and begin protocol procedures in the early hours of treatment of decompensation. A discussion regarding ED policy and a plan for shared research responsibility will be necessary if research interventions will be occurring in that setting.

Funding support from National Heart, Lung, Blood Institute.
The author has nothing to disclose.
Duke University Box 3693, Durham, NC 27710, USA
E-mail address: patricia.adams@duke.edu

Heart Failure Clin 7 (2011) 545–551
doi:10.1016/j.hfc.2011.06.006

Characteristics of the Coordinating Team

The qualifications and experience of the members of the heart failure SBR coordinating team are crucial to the operation of the clinical trials. To ensure the quality and integrity of the studies, the team needs a lead coordinator who understands the scientific, legal, institutional, financial, and ethical issues and a team of professional, well-educated, skilled staff members.[6] Coordinators for acute heart failure clinical trials need the usual skills required of coordinators: attention to detail, organization skills, ability to understand the research design, and implementation of protocol. In addition, the CRCs engaged in acute heart failure trials need clinical, teaching, and presentation skills unique to managing clinical trials of acute heart failure.

The clinical skills necessary include nursing assessment, physical assessment, intravenous (IV) therapy administration, monitoring ability, awareness of side effects, and knowledge of standard therapies for acute heart failure, standard operating procedures, and unit policies for the nursing care of patients with acute heart failure. The coordinators need these special skills to successfully comply with the protocol and simultaneously assist in managing the subject's medical therapy.[7]

An emerging nursing career path is a transition from nurse clinical specialist to CRC.[8] Recruiting nurse CRCs with previous cardiology unit, intensive care unit, coronary care unit, and heart failure specialist experiences is especially advantageous for the heart failure research team. These coordinators possess the knowledge, skills, and appropriate licensure to identify appropriate participants and perform protocol procedures for acute heart failure trials.[9]

Teaching, presentation, and communication skills are important assets for heart failure CRCs. Coordinators present the trial design and procedures to multidisciplinary teams, patients, and families. They may be teaching the care team members new or modified therapies, such as experimental medications with unique side effects and new or modified methods of assessing and recording observations that are end points in the clinical trials. Examples of new or modified assessments include visual analog scale dyspnea scores, a urine collection that requires special handling, teaching the care team members the importance of and method for collecting data for assessments, or events that take place when the CRC is not present.

Capacity Planning and Budgeting

The heart failure SBR has the capacity to operate multiple clinical trials simultaneously. The capacity depends on several variables, including the available personnel, complexity of the protocol, access to the appropriate cohort of potential subjects, availability of devices, and health system policies regarding processes and procedures. These same variables are factors that determine the study budget.

Access to the appropriate cohort of potential subjects is critical to the feasibility of the study. Hospital census figures are useful in predicting admission rates and diagnoses and may be used in research with adherence to Human Research Protection Program policies. A particularly useful tool is an online query tool to access hospital information. The tool, when queried accurately, produces a report of historic data about the potential cohort. If the available cohort is large, enrollment can be expected to be brisk and personnel use will be maximized. If the cohort is small and enrollment is infrequent, a larger amount of personnel time will be spent in screening. Both scenarios should be reflected in the budget.

Protocol complexity affects both the capacity and budget. Many assessments of acute heart failure therapy, such as vital signs, daily weight, intake, and output, are standard-of-care (SOC) assessments. The frequency varies based on patient acuity and nursing unit policy. Collaboration with nursing unit managers in reviewing protocols provides an opportunity to prospectively evaluate who will perform the assessments as SOC and which assessments will be performed by the research staff. Assessments performed by research staff on off hours and weekends may incur higher cost and may result in the need for additional staff.

Close collaboration with the clinical enterprise and nurse managers also reveals unit/hospital policy pertaining to the use of an investigational drug service, the availability of and procedure for using device therapies such as ultrafiltration, extended length catheters, central lines for certain medications, and specialty teams such as intravenous or peripherally inserted central catheter line teams. All these aspects affect resource use and, therefore, capacity and budget.

The current length of stay (LOS) for acute heart failure is 4.3 days,[10,11] so inevitably there will be protocol interventions and assessments that take place on the weekend. There is also a need for the clinical care team to have access to the coordinator and PI for questions regarding the protocol on a 24/7 basis. Financing and scheduling for this procedure will have an impact on the study budget. Using a team approach with a portfolio of trials, the heart failure SBR unit has the flexibility needed to accommodate this variation in workload. It has been our experience that a team of 3 trained heart failure nurse CRCs rotating on-call and on weekend coverage is probably the minimum necessary to avoid coordinator burnout.

Armed with the information mentioned earlier, the lead coordinator and faculty medical director are able to plan the deployment of resources. The portfolio of trials can be built that are complementary to one another, which maximizes screening and recruiting effort. For example, one trial is for recruiting subjects with low ejection fraction, one for patients with preserved function, one trial for recruiting within the first 24 hours, and one for enrolling subjects with renal dysfunction after 48 hours. A portfolio of 2 to 4 actively enrolling trials of acute heart failure is appropriate to operate the SBR efficiently.

CHALLENGES IN CONDUCTING CLINICAL TRIALS IN ACUTE HEART FAILURE
Recruitment Challenges

In a busy clinical environment with rotating multidisciplinary teams, it is challenging to keep everyone informed of the details of currently enrolling clinical trials. In the recently conducted before and after study of research attitude, Dale and colleagues[12] reported no differences for clinicians' preawareness and postawareness campaign. The campaign consisted of prominently displayed posters and an informational pamphlet. Response for clinicians was not statically significant with 36% at baseline and 33% postintervention. Despite the single center and small size of the study, it underscores the importance of CRC physical presence with the clinical teams to enhance recruitment.

A physical presence during morning rounds is the most successful recruitment strategy for acute heart failure. This is, however, a time-consuming strategy. The coordinator arrives fully prepared but must await the appropriate opportunity to discuss the potential subject. The order of the rounding team is subject to the acuity of the assigned patients, discharge deadlines, training opportunities, and meeting schedules. The coordinator often needs to communicate with multiple rounding teams on multiple nursing units. A well-organized approach is highly desirable, and often a colleague is necessary. Because of the unpredictable nature of this screening workload, a team approach is useful.

Even with a team approach, there is opportunity to miss potential subjects. Patients with acute heart failure will be admitted 7 days a week. In a recent study by Fonarow and colleagues,[13] examining day of admission and discharge in the OPTIMIZE-HF data, the highest percentage of admissions occurred on Monday; they were evenly distributed from Tuesday through Friday, with Saturday and Sunday being less frequent. If, because of coordinator schedules, screening is not possible 7 days a week, then screening Monday through Friday will maximize the effort with a loss of only 22% on the weekend.

The opposite problem to that of missing patients is the problem of patients being recruited for multiple clinical trials simultaneously. The portfolio approach to clinical trials can lead to a situation in which a patient is the potential subject in multiple acute heart failure clinical trials. Patients with acute heart failure have multiple comorbid conditions for which there are competing clinical trials. Nursing research also competes for recruitment of patients with acute heart failure. Potential conflicts occur with drug-drug and drug-device interventions. Trials that might be complementary are trials of a drug or device combined with a trial of heart failure education modalities or heart failure behavior modification studies. Coenrollment in clinical trials can be accommodated with careful communication between coordinators, PIs, the clinical care team, and the sponsors. It is recommended when planning coenrollment that the coordinators of both trials plan interventions, questionnaires, and follow-up visits to minimize subject fatigue. It is also recommended that written contact information be provided to the subject to prevent confusion between studies.

Retention Challenges

Subject retention is vital to the collection of end point data in clinical trials. Acute heart failure trials usually have short follow-up schedules and, therefore, are not subject to the volunteer fatigue associated with the multiple follow-up visits that occur in outpatient studies with years-long follow-up. However, there are some occasions that present challenges for the coordinators.

Instances in which the subject withdraws from participation are rare but do occur. Subjects who are fatigued with dyspnea and agree to participate because it is the course of least resistance may change their mind when more rested. Family members who were not present during the consent process may express concern and/or disagreement with their loved one's decision to participate. Most of these challenges can be met with a thoughtful and sensitive consent process, for example, interspersing rest periods during the consent discussion and calling family member who are not able to be present. Coordinators may need to repeat parts of the consent process with infinite patience to subjects whose fatigue interferes with their ability to pay attention or comprehend. The coordinators may need to spend extra time with family members who have additional questions.

Subjects may grow weary of the intervention and may request to withdraw either from the intervention or from the study. An experienced nurse clinical coordinator will engage the care team to identify the aspect of the intervention that is most troublesome to the patient and brainstorm a solution. For example, a patient with an additional dedicated intravenous line for study drug infusion may have more freedom of motion if the intravenous pole is relocated or a patient weary of the connection to an ultrafiltration device might be more comfortable in a recliner. Careful listening and creative problem solving may enable the patient to continue to participate.

A more challenging aspect of retention occurs when subjects enroll in a research study of acute heart failure at a tertiary care center and are unable or unwilling to return for follow-up visits owing to time and distance. This prospect must be discussed during the consent process. If a suitable arrangement cannot be agreed on, an alternative research study with phone call follow-up may be more appropriate for that subject.

Data Collection and Protocol Compliance Challenges

The patients who have been recruited and retained in clinical studies deserve utmost respect for their volunteer contribution. It is extremely important to honor their contribution with accurate and thorough collection of all data. Much of the data collected will be part of the SOC for patients hospitalized with acute heart failure. For example, daily weight, intake and output, vital signs, and oxygen saturation are clinical assessments for which there are standard institutional procedures that produce objective, accurate, and replicable data. These types of data are subject to the recording accuracy or omissions of the clinical care team. It is important that the research team uses a strategy of trust but verify. The team should trust that the SOC is followed but verify with sufficient frequency to avoid omission of end point data.

Assessments such as dyspnea, fatigue, and overall well-being are subjective assessments, which rely heavily on the clinical training and experience of the nursing staff.[14,15] Some investigators recommend hiring a coordinator to oversee every detail of data collection. Stone[16] writes "It appears that hospitals in many areas are slashing their staff as part of their cost-cutting efforts. The result is more harried staff and more medical errors. It's bad enough when any error happens with patients; it can be personally and professionally devastating if it happens during a clinical trial." In support of dedicated research staff, Travers stated, "Data collection by nurses and physicians who are working shifts is hard. They are busy with their first priority which is patient care."[17]

As desirable as it might be to hire a coordinator to oversee every detail, in the case of research involving acute heart failure, many of the assessments take place around the clock and the cost would be prohibitive. This dilemma needs to be addressed because more often clinical research and care take place concurrently in the same system.[4] A compromise is for the PI, study team, and clinical team to review and assess the specific protocol assessments and determine which are essential and feasible to be done by the coordinator for accuracy, consistency, and reliability and which can be delegated carefully to the clinical care team. Imperative proactive steps are communication with the nurse management leaders and clinical educators. Clinical staff education should include the importance of the data collection, need for accuracy, and importance of the contribution the clinical staff is making toward improving patient's outcomes.

To improve communication, protocol compliance, and data collection, coordinators can establish frequent contact with the clinical team, including evening and weekend hours and provision of a 24/7 contact number. Developing a strong collaboration between the research staff and the clinical staff requires consistent, persistent, ongoing dialogue and the support of the clinical and institutional leadership. Rapport, trust, and partnership will be built by coordinators who make the effort to be present daily and to talk with the staff nurses.[18] The nurse coordinator is in a unique position to express empathy and appreciation for the clinical staff and to provide education of the clinical care team members.

Educating clinical staff has many benefits. The clinical care nurse who understands the protocol may suggest potential candidates to the research nurse,[19] thereby increasing enrollment. Clinical care nurses will be able to help respond to questions raised by patients or their families, which aides in retention. They can also assist in supporting and educating fellow staff members[20] to improve protocol compliance and data collection.

There are many opportunities and models for staff education. Staff in-service can be done in groups, such as during change of shift and in mini-sessions during break periods. Online training can be established on a staff intranet, and power point presentations can be sent via email. Offering education credit can provide incentives for staff participation. Perhaps the most effective training occurs one-to-one with the nurse providing care to the patient enrolled in the trial. Providing instructions orally, in writing, at the bedside, and in a resource binder on the unit all labeled with the research team pager provides the care teams with resources to answer their questions as needed and improve protocol adherence and data collection.

Clinical Decision Making Versus Protocol-Driven Care

As inpatients are enrolled in clinical trials, there will be many questions posed by the medical care team regarding clinical decision making and the effect the protocol may have on clinical care. Within the heart failure SBR, the PIs and their colleagues will be familiar with the research protocols and their relationship to clinical care. However, many patients with acute heart failure who are eligible to enroll will be in the service of providers who are less familiar with the protocols. An experienced clinically knowledgeable coordinator with specialization in heart failure who understands the protocol will be able to round with the care team, answer questions, and refer to the PI as appropriate. This additive bridge between the clinical enterprise and clinical research facilitates the research while providing the best possible clinical care for the patient.

The Equipoise Challenge

Equipoise is an important concept in research. As defined by Freeman,[21] equipoise is a state of genuine uncertainty on the part of the clinical investigator regarding the comparative therapeutic merits of each arm in a trial. If not present, equipoise can present a challenge to enrollment,[22] retention, and compliance with procedures. The individual members of the multidisciplinary care teams may have personal or professional experiences, which leave them without equipoise regarding the study intervention. Even patients may think that they do not have equipoise about the clinical trial.

Nurses have a role that is defined as patient protector and advocate.[19,23] Nurses may believe that the patient is vulnerable because of high acuity, fatigue, or shortness of breath,[7] or they may express concern due to the burden of study interventions.[18]

Continuing education regarding the treatment of acute heart failure; the current Heart Failure Society of America (HFSA), American College of Cardiology, and American Heart Association guidelines; and current research or lack of research can help the clinical teams understand the protocol and the questions being asked. Topics of discussion should also include what clinical research is and what makes it ethical.[24] This is an opportunity for a joint effort by the PI and the nurse coordinators to share information that will help others understand the research. Close working relationships between the clinical teams and the research teams will foster the knowledge, competence, advocacy, and creativity necessary to maintain the balance between research and patient protection.[24]

Occasionally, patients state that they are certain they know the answer to the research question and describe themselves as without equipoise. An example might be a patient who is invited to participate in a study of the route of diuretic administration. The patient may have experienced previous success with IV bolus diuretic on several occasions and less relief with continuous administration on a different occasion. He or she may or may not know the dose but is certain of the route of administration. In this case, there may be a different research study for which the patient might be a more appropriate candidate and about which he or she might have equipoise.

The Challenge of Role Clarity from the Patient Perspective

The blending of the clinical enterprise and research creates a team with overlapping roles. The distinction between the nurse as a caregiver and the nurse as a researcher may not be appreciated by the patient.[24] Nurse coordinators may encounter situations in which their clinical expertise is called upon outside the boundaries of the protocol. An example might be the coordinator of a diuretic therapy trial who participates in clinical rounds during a discussion of heart transplant with the subject enrolled in the diuretic trial. Afterward, the patient may question the coordinator about the benefit of transplant. Experience, mentoring, and open dialogue with managers and investigators are essential elements in helping nurse coordinators navigate the ethics of situations such as this.[25]

The clinical care/research team that rounds together plans together, and this benefits the research subjects with opportunities and attention. Care must be taken to help patients understand the procedures and assessments that are specific to the protocol and those that are part of their clinical care. After rounds, the coordinators will need to reinforce the details, for example, explain to patients that the echocardiogram ordered for the day is part of their clinical care and the 24-hour urine collection is part of the research.

LOS Challenge

Decreasing hospital LOS and reducing rehospitalizations are improvements in outcome that are priorities of the health care system and a goal of clinical research in heart failure. There is anecdotal reporting that participation in research adds to LOS because of the additional time to consent, randomize, receive specialized study product from a research pharmacy, and delay of diagnostic procedures to complete study procedures. A search of the literature does not indicate that participation in research while hospitalized with acute heart failure increases LOS. The median LOS in the ASCEND (Acute Study of Clinical Effectiveness of Nesiritide in Decompensated Heart Failure) trial for sites in North America is 4 days, which approximates the median LOS in the ADHERE (Acute Decompensated Heart Failure National) registry, which was 4.3 days.[11]

The Challenge of Newly Published Research that Affects Ongoing Research

During a clinical trial, the publication of results from other investigations can have a profound effect on the trial underway. Reduction in hospital readmission rates for patients with heart failure is an important objective. The HFSA 2010 guidelines[1] recommend a return to clinic (RTC) visit within 2 weeks of discharge. This guideline is supported in the recently published research of Hernandez and colleagues,[26] who concluded that "Patients who are discharged from hospitals that have higher early follow-up rates have a lower risk of 30-day readmission." This has created a dilemma for current research studies in acute heart failure with a planned protocol visit at 30 days. Subjects who have made an RTC visit at 2 weeks postdischarge do not wish to return 2 weeks later for the 30-day protocol visit. At the time the protocol was written, the research

Table 1
Research challenges and solutions

Challenges	Solutions
Recruitment challenges	
Protocol awareness	Coordinator presence on units and with rounding teams
Recruiting schedule	Recruit Monday through Friday if unable to include Saturday and Sunday
Competing enrollment	Careful coenrollment, planning, and communication with other research teams
Retention challenges	
Withdrawal	Thoughtful and sensitive consent process to minimize the occurrence; include rest periods, family members, and repetition as needed
Withdrawal from intervention	Engage the clinical care team to help listen carefully and to creatively solve problems
Protocol and data collection challenges	
SOC data	Trust but verify
Subjective assessments	Assess who should be responsible; carefully train; and reinforce the rationale, method, and importance
Clinical decision making versus protocol-driven care	
Questions posed by clinicians	Coordinator available to round with the team and serve as a bridge between clinical care and research
Equipoise	
If missing from care team and/or nurses	Opportunity for investigators and coordinators to share in discussion with care team members of current guidelines, research, therapies, and ethics
If missing from patient	Offer the opportunity to consider participation in a different research study
Role clarity	
Nurse as caregiver/researcher	Provide mentors, experience, and dialogue with investigators to navigate ethics
Clinical care team/research team	Reinforce as necessary which procedures are clinical and which are research

and subsequent guidelines had not been published. This can be expected to resolve as the current trials come to completion and new protocols are written with the newer guidelines in mind.

The challenges and solutions discussed here are summarized in **Table 1**.

SUMMARY

The model of a heart failure SBR unit with responsibility for conducting multiple clinical trials of acute heart failure has the advantage of stability and a structure with personnel who have the training, experience, support, and skills to align with the clinical enterprise to produce ethical reliable research that will improve understanding of acute heart failure and improve clinical care. The many challenges of conducting clinical trials in acute heart failure can be addressed with education, collaboration, training, and skill development within the SBR structure.

REFERENCES

1. Liindenfeld J, Albert NM, Boehmer JP, et al. HFSA 2010 comprehensive heart failure practice guideline. J Card Fail 2010;16(6):e1–194.
2. Yusuf S, Bosch J, Devereaux PJ, et al. Sensible guidelines for the conduct of large randomized trials. Clin Trials 2008;5(1):38–9.
3. Califf RM, Harrington RA, Madre LK, et al. Curbing the cardiovascular disease epidemic: aligning industry, government, payers, and academics. Health Aff (Millwood) 2007;26(1):62–74.
4. Califf RM. Clinical research sites—the underappreciated component of the clinical research system. JAMA 2009;302(18):2025–7.
5. Collins SP, Levy PD, Lindsell CJ, et al. The rationale for an acute heart failure syndromes clinical trials network. J Card Fail 2009;15(6):467–74.
6. Jones C, Harrison L, Carter S, et al. Education and training preferences of clinical research managers. Res Pract 2008;9(6):202–11.
7. Jairath N, Ulrich CM, Ley C. Ethical considerations in the recruitment of research subjects from hospitalized, cardiovascular patient populations. J Cardiovasc Nurs 2005;20(1):56–61.
8. Shields A, LaRue EM. Transitioning from clinician to clinical research coordinator. Am J Nurs 2010; 110(Suppl 1):26–7.
9. Baer A, Bechar N, Cohen G, et al. Basic steps to building a research program. J Oncol Pract 2010;6(1):45–7.
10. Velis E, Whiteman AS, Caballero GS, et al. Congestive heart failure admissions: factors related to hospital length of stay. J Med Pract Manage 2008;23(6):350–7.
11. Adams KF, Fonarow GC, Emerman CL, et al. Characteristics and outcomes of patients hospitalized for heart failure in the United States: rationale, design,

and preliminary observations from the first 100,000 cases in the Acute Decompensated Heart Failure National Registry (ADHERE). Am Heart J 2005; 149(2):209–16.
12. Dale C, Fowler RA, Adhikari NK, et al. Implementation of a research awareness program in the critical care unit: effects on families and clinicians. Intensive Crit Care Nurs 2010;26(2):69–74.
13. Fonarow GC, Abraham WT, Albert NM, et al. Day of admission and clinical outcomes for patients hospitalized for heart failure: findings from the Organized Program to Initiate Lifesaving Treatment in Hospitalized Patients With Heart Failure (OPTIMIZE-HF). Circ Heart Fail 2008;1(1):50–7.
14. Phipps WJ, Sands JK, Marek JF, et al. Medical-surgical nursing: concepts and clinical practice. St Louis (MO): Mosby; 1999.
15. Davis L. Cardiovascular nursing secrets: [your cardiovascular questions answered by experts you trust]. St Louis (MO): Elsevier Mosby; 2004.
16. Stone J. How to adapt to the changing clinical trial climate—CTN best practices. Clinical trials networks best practices. Available at: https://www.ctnbestpractices.org/second-opinions/how-to-adapt-to-the-changing-clinical-trial-climate. Accessed August 28, 2010.
17. Boost bottom line with research nurse. ED Manag 2001;13(12):140–2.
18. Chlan L, Guttormson J, Tracy MF, et al. Strategies for overcoming site and recruitment challenges in research studies based in intensive care units. Am J Crit Care 2009;18(5):410–7.
19. Poston RD, Buescher CR. The essential role of the clinical research nurse (CRN). Urol Nurs 2010; 30(1):55–63, 77.
20. CR education should extend to clinical care nursing staff: efforts can help with patient recruitment. Clinical Trials Administrator 2010;8(1):10–1.
21. Freedman B. Equipoise and the ethics of clinical research. N Engl J Med 1987;317(3):141–5.
22. Frye RL, Simari RD, Gersh BJ, et al. Ethical issues in cardiovascular research involving humans. Circulation 2009;120(21):2113–21.
23. NursingWorld. Code of ethics. Available at: http://nursingworld.org/ethics/code/protected_nwcoe629.htm#3.3. Accessed August 28, 2010.
24. Grady C, Edgerly M. Science, technology, and innovation: nursing responsibilities in clinical research. Nurs Clin North Am 2009;44(4):471–81.
25. Wilkes L, Cert R, Beale B. Role conflict: appropriateness of a nurse researcher's actions in the clinical field. Nurse Res 2005;12(4):57–70.
26. Hernandez AF, Greiner MA, Fonarow GC, et al. Relationship between early physician follow-up and 30-day readmission among Medicare beneficiaries hospitalized for heart failure. JAMA 2010;303(17): 1716–22.

Pharmacogenetics in Heart Failure Trials

Mona Fiuzat, PharmD[a],*, Michael R. Bristow, MD, PhD[b]

KEYWORDS

- Pharmacogenetics • Adrenergic receptors • Heart failure
- Clinical trials

Personalized medicine is a growing theme in clinical trials and research initiatives, stimulated by a variety of factors including funding opportunities supported by government agencies, a need for novel therapeutic approaches, and a growing body of literature linking genetic variation to clinical outcomes. Personalized medicine is fundamentally about obtaining information from an individual's genome and using it to make therapeutic decisions tailored to the individual. A natural starting point for personalized medicine is pharmacogenetics: using genetic information to predict an individual's response to therapy, both in terms of efficacy and safety.

In oncology, the therapeutic index of anti-cancer agents can, in some settings, be improved by pharmacogenetic targeting.[1–5] In human immunodeficiency virus, pharmacogenetic markers can be used to predict drug safety.[6] As knowledge of appropriate use and clinical usefulness of companion genetic testing matures, pharmacogenetic strategies can be incorporated into therapeutic guidelines.

In cardiology, genetic variations have been associated with hydroxy-methylglutaryl coenzyme A (HMG CoA) reductase inhibitors (statins), where genetic variants can help identify patients more likely to experience adverse effects.[7] Variations in cytochrome P450 genes may alter an individual's ability to metabolize drugs. In cardiology, this is highly relevant to anticoagulant and antithrombotic therapies, and may increase bleeding risk in certain patients. In August 2007, the US Food and Drug Administration approved revision of warfarin labeling to include genetic testing,[8] because 2 genetic variants predict response to therapy.[9] The VKORC1 allele predicts sensitivity to warfarin, and the cytochrome P450 2C9 gene variant predicts drug metabolism. Genetic variation has also been linked to clinical outcomes, such as the increased risk of ventricular arrhythmias and sudden cardiac death in patients with a β2 adrenergic receptor (AR) polymorphism.[10] Advances in technology and the ability to perform genome-wide association studies (GWAS) have increased our knowledge base and, in a short time, these studies have identified genetic determinants of disease risk in several therapeutic areas, including diabetes,[11–14] hyperlipidemia,[15–17] and atherosclerosis.[18,19]

HEART FAILURE

Heart failure is a major and growing public health problem, with more than 5 million people in the United States living with chronic heart failure, 550,000 new cases diagnosed each year, and approximately 300,000 deaths caused by heart failure.[20] A variety of demographic trends, including the aging of the population and greater survival after acute myocardial infarction, suggest that the prevalence of heart failure is likely to continue increasing.[21] Although there have been significant advances in the treatment of heart failure, there is a substantial need for greater targeting of heart failure therapy. Morbidity and mortality from heart failure remain high despite the improvements in therapy. Pharmacologic regimens have become increasingly complex, and standard heart failure therapy now frequently consists of 5 or more drugs. The economic impact of chronic heart failure

Disclosures: Fiuzat, shareholder, ARCA biopharma; Bristow, CEO and cofounder, ARCA biopharma.
[a] Duke University Medical Center, 2400 Pratt Street, Room 8011, Durham, NC 27710, USA
[b] ARCA biopharma, Division of Cardiology, University of Colorado Health Sciences Center, Denver, CO, USA
* Corresponding author.
E-mail address: mona.fiuzat@duke.edu

Heart Failure Clin 7 (2011) 553–559
doi:10.1016/j.hfc.2011.06.010

hospitalizations is approximately $35 billion annually in the United States alone. Greater targeting of therapy would allow the focused use of drugs most likely to be efficacious and safe in individual patients, potentially enhancing compliance and improving outcomes.

PHARMACOGENETICS IN HEART FAILURE TRIALS
Polymorphisms of the β-ARs

β-blockers are one of the cornerstones of chronic heart failure therapy, with substantial impact on mortality and morbidity. However, β-blocker therapy is not efficacious, or is poorly tolerated, in some patients with heart failure, making this a logical possibility for genetically targeted therapy. The β1-AR position 389 Arg/Gly polymorphism, caused by a nucleotide 1165 C (Arg) to G (Gly) transversion, has been widely studied. The β1 389 Arg/Gly polymorphism alters signaling in multiple models, and may affect the β-blocker therapeutic response in heart failure.[22]

Studies have suggested that the β1 389 AR Arg/Gly polymorphism may have an impact on left ventricular ejection fraction improvement (LVEF) with β-blocker therapy,[23–27] but these studies have had several limitations and are not conclusive for clinical usefulness. Many smaller studies have examined this polymorphism, with conflicting results regarding the impact on disease risk, progression, and response to treatment.[28–30]

Two large (phase III) randomized, placebo-controlled heart failure trials with β-blockers,

MERIT-HF, and the β-Blocker Evaluation of Survival Trial (BEST), included DNA substudies. The β1 389 Arg/Gly polymorphism was evaluated in both studies. The Metoprolol CR/XL Randomized Intervention Trial in Heart Failure (MERIT-HF) contained a 600-patient substudy testing the hypothesis that the β1 389 AR Arg/Gly polymorphism influenced the outcome of heart failure, or conferred a differential response to treatment with Metoprolol CR/XL.[31] Based on previous studies, the MERIT-HF substudy hypothesized that patients with the β1-389 AR Gly variant would have better outcomes, as measured by mortality and hospitalization. The investigators further hypothesized that patients with the β1-389 AR Arg allele would show a greater response to treatment with β-blockade. In this study, no effect of the polymorphism was observed in either a morbidity/mortality benefit or a response to metoprolol treatment.

In contrast, BEST showed a significant impact of the β1 389 AR Arg/Gly polymorphism on response to treatment with the β-blocker bucindolol. BEST contained a 1040-patient DNA substudy, evaluating improvement in morbidity/mortality by β1 AR genotype.[22] Patients who were β1 389 AR Arg homozygotes had significant improvements in cause-specific and all-cause morbidity and mortality compared with patients who were β1 389 AR Gly carriers. Fig. 1 gives Kaplan-Meier curves for bucindolol or placebo in the β1 Arg/Arg or Gly carrier genotypes for the combined endpoint of all-cause mortality or heart failure hospitalization. For patients with the Arg/Arg genotype, there is a substantial (33%, hazard ratio

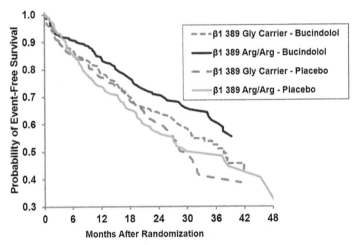

Subpop	Group 1 Event Rate	Group 2 Event Rate	HR and CI	P value
Bucindolol Treatment	Arg/Arg 87/257 (34%)	Gly Carrier 105/258 (41%)	0.77 (0.57 – 1.03)	.08
Placebo Treatment	Arg/Arg 102/236 (43%)	Gly Carrier 131/289 (45%)	0.99 (0.76 – 1.30)	.95
Arg/Arg Genotype	Bucindolol 87/259 (34%)	Placebo 102/236 (43%)	0.67 (0.50 – 0.89)	.005
Gly Carrier Genotype	Bucindolol 105/258 (41%)	Placebo 131/289 (45%)	0.86 (0.66 – 1.11)	.24

Fig. 1. All-cause mortality/heart failure hospitalization, BEST Trial DNA substudy.

0.67, $P = .005$) reduction in the event rate in the bucindolol compared with the placebo group. In contrast, patients with Gly genotypes (Gly carriers) do not have a significant efficacy effect (hazard ratio 0.86, $P = .24$). There was no difference in outcomes for placebo-treated patients based on genotype (hazard ratio 0.99), indicating that this polymorphism does not influence disease progression within the time frame of the BEST clinical trial, which had a mean follow-up of 2 years.[22] Because the BEST trial was unique in many of its enrollment criteria, which led to an advanced clinical heart failure population that was enriched in African Americans, the apparently unique effects of bucindolol on $\beta 1$ 389 Arg/Gly polymorphisms compared with the effects of metoprolol CR/XL in MERIT-HF could have been caused by patient selection. However, when the BEST trial had the enrollment criteria adjusted[32] to that for the other major β-blocker heart failure mortality trials (COPERNICUS, MERIT-HF, and CIBIS-II), the enhanced effect of bucindolol in the $\beta 1$ 389 Arg/Arg versus Gly carrier genotype is even more pronounced (**Fig. 2**). In this subgroup the reduction in the combined endpoint of mortality/heart failure hospitalization in the Arg/Arg genotype was 42% ($P = .004$), compared with 4% ($P = .80$) in Gly carriers. Therefore the $\beta 1$ 389 Arg/Gly pharmacogenetic effects of bucindolol seem to be caused

by unique pharmacologic properties of the drug, and not to differences in the patients enrolled in the BEST versus MERIT-HF or other trials.

Another recent study of 637 patients with heart failure evaluated the outcomes of patients treated with the β-blocker metoprolol succinate or carvedilol by $\beta 1$ 389 AR genotype.[30] This trial showed no impact of the $\beta 1$ 389 Arg/Gly polymorphism on survival in patients treated with either metoprolol or carvedilol, supporting the findings from the MERIT-HF substudy and leading to the hypothesis that there may be a drug-specific interaction of the β-blocker bucindolol that may not occur with metoprolol or carvedilol. One plausible explanation for this is the unique pharmacology of bucindolol, because it selectively leads to the inactivation of constitutively active (R*) $\beta 1$ ARs.[33] In isolated failing human heart preparations genotyped as $\beta 1$ AR 389 Arg/Arg, bucindolol was an inverse agonist, which indicates R* receptors shifting to an inactive state, whereas metoprolol and carvedilol were neutral antagonists.[22,33] Another unique pharmacologic mechanism of bucindolol, its norepinephrine (NE)-lowering or sympatholytic properties, may also contribute to an enhanced effect on $\beta 1$ 389 Arg receptors, which have a higher affinity for NE than the Gly variant.[34]

Other polymorphisms identified to have potential heart failure associations have also yielded

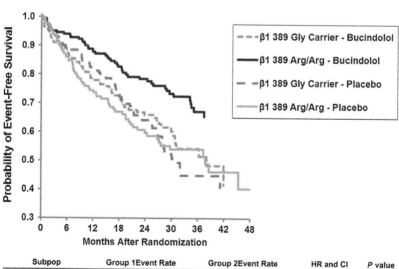

Subpop	Group 1 Event Rate	Group 2 Event Rate	HR and CI	P value
Bucindolol Treatment	Arg/Arg 48/174 (28%)	Gly Carrier 62/155 (40%)	0.59 (0.40 – 0.87)	.007
Placebo Treatment	Arg/Arg 69/162 (43%)	Gly Carrier 74/171 (43%)	1.02 (0.73 – 1.42)	.909
Arg/Arg Genotype	Bucindolol 48/174 (28%)	Placebo 69/162 (43%)	0.58 (0.40 – 0.84)	.004
Gly Carrier Genotype	Bucindolol 62/155 (40%)	Placebo 74/171 (43%)	0.96 (0.68 – 1.35)	.797

Fig. 2. All-cause mortality/heart failure hospitalization, BEST Trial DNA substudy by subgroup matching patient characteristics. (*Adapted from* Domanski M, Kraus-Steinrauf H, Massie M, et al. A comparative analysis of the results from 4 trials of beta-blocker therapy for heart failure: BEST, CIBIS-II, MERIT-HF, and COPERNICUS. J Card Fail 2003;9(5):354–63.)

inconsistent or limited data. In addition to the β1 389 gene variant, the β1 49 Ser/Gly polymorphism has shown some effect on response to β-blockers; however, studies have been underpowered and shown inconsistent associations.[24,30,35,36]

Potentially important polymorphisms studied in the β2 AR include the β2 16 Arg/Gly and β2 27 Gln/Gly gene variants, but these also have not shown a consistent association with drug response or outcomes.[22–24,30,37]

Polymorphisms in the Renin-Angiotensin-Aldosterone System

DNA substudy information is available from 2 additional heart failure trials. The African American Heart Failure Trial (AHeFT) evaluated the addition of fixed combination isosorbide dinitrates and hydralazine versus placebo to standard heart failure therapy. AHeFT contained a DNA substudy, the Genetic Risk Assessment of Heart Failure in African Americans (GRAHF), designed to evaluate polymorphisms identified in mostly white patients to evaluate outcomes in a black heart failure population, and to identify whether or not the apparent racial difference in response could be explained by genetic factors.[38] In this substudy of black patients with heart failure, the aldosterone synthase gene (CYP11B2) position 344 T/C polymorphism was evaluated. The TT genotype was associated with better event-free survival and response to therapy with isosorbide dinitrates and hydralazine than C allele carriers, with CC homozygotes having the poorest event-free survival.

The Candesartan in Heart Failure, Assessment of Mortality and Morbidity Trial (CHARM) collected DNA samples on a subset of patients. In an exploratory proof-of-concept study in 31 of these patients, 10 genetic polymorphisms were examined.[39] Of these, genetic variation in the angiotensin II type 1 receptor (AGTR1) A1166C was linked to an interaction with candesartan treatment response. Patients who were AA homozygous appeared more sensitive to treatment, suggesting that patients carrying the C allele may benefit from higher doses of candesartan. In addition, this gene variant may affect the degree of left ventricular remodeling with angiotensin II receptor blockers (ARBs).[39–41] Although these exploratory studies have limitations with small sample sizes, they may suggest a candidate gene association for future studies with ARBs.

Several other genetic polymorphisms have been evaluated in smaller heart failure trials. The angiotensin-converting enzyme (ACE) gene insertion versus deletion (I/D) polymorphism has been widely studied.[40,42–45] The Genetic Risk Assessment of Cardiac Events (GRACE) was a single-center, 328-patient trial examining the ACE I/D polymorphism influence on β-blocker or ACE inhibitor response.[43,44] Data from GRACE indicated that patients who were ACE DD homozygotes had an increased risk of death or cardiac transplant compared with the ACE II or ID genotypes. Furthermore, patients with the ACE DD genotype had significantly better response to β-blockers than the II or ID genotype cohort.[43] The ACE DD homozygous patients also appeared to benefit from higher doses of ACE inhibitors versus a low dose of ACE inhibitor therapy.[44] This important study suggests that treatment selection and dosing may be associated with this genetic variation; however, the data have been inconsistent and require further investigation.[40,42,45,46]

Polymorphisms and Exercise in Heart Failure

A nonpharmacologic and nondevice therapy routinely used for cardiology patients is exercise. Exercise capacity (as judged by 6-minute walk and cardiopulmonary exercise testing) is a known predictor of morbidity and mortality in cardiac patients.[47] Recently, a large trial evaluating the impact of exercise therapy in patients with heart failure was reported.[48] The Efficacy and Safety of Exercise Training as a Treatment Modality in Patients with Chronic Heart Failure Trial (HF-ACTION) collected DNA samples on a subset of patients, and the DNA substudy will be the first to evaluate genetic variations that may affect response or adherence to lifestyle intervention in a large heart failure trial. Although β2 AR polymorphisms do not seem to affect outcomes with drug therapy,[30] there is evidence of a potential association with response to exercise.[49–51] In patients with heart failure, the β216 Arg/Gly, β2 27 Gln/Gly, and β2 164 Thr/Ile may potentially affect response to exercise.[49,52] Previously reported data also show potential interaction with the ACE D/I polymorphisms.[53,54] In a 57-patient study, the ACE DD polymorphism was associated with decreased exercise tolerance in patients with heart failure.[54] The results of the HF-ACTION DNA substudy will provide important information on whether or not these polymorphisms influence long-term outcomes with exercise training, and may provide insight to the patients who may benefit most from lifestyle intervention.

Polymorphisms and Devices in Heart Failure

Genetic polymorphisms have also been investigated as potential tools to select patients who might benefit from implantable cardiac defibrillators (ICDs). The β1 389 AR Arg/Gly, GNB3 C825

T, GP IIb/IIIa PI[A1]/PI[A2], and transforming growth factor-β have been identified as possible predictors of ICD response,[55–57] providing an important approach given the high cost of therapy.

Biventricular (BIV) pacing has emerged as another area of heart failure therapy that shows potential for genetic targeting. At least 1 ongoing trial is testing the hypothesis that genetic polymorphisms influence the incidence and degree of response to BIV pacing in heart failure.[54]

SUMMARY

There is ongoing research evaluating many other potential pharmacogenetic targets in heart failure. Several challenges exist despite the potential benefits. Genome-wide studies may identify an association of a gene variant with pathogenesis of disease, but biologically plausible explanations should exist for the association. For candidate gene targets, the polymorphism must be functionally relevant, prevalent, and provide potential for therapeutic intervention. Selection bias may exist in clinical trial cohorts, and may not represent the true population at risk. In these studies, sample sizes have been small or modest at best, and rigorous statistical testing with multiple comparisons has not been systematically and consistently applied. In addition, questions remain on the level of evidence needed to support product approval or labeling.

It is estimated that in the next year nearly 300,000 patients will die, and 1 million patients will be hospitalized, because of heart failure.[20] High annual mortality, high morbidity, and heterogeneity of response to treatment underscore the need for predictability of response in this patient population. Although prime time testing and application of pharmacogenetics is not currently being used in heart failure, we believe this treatment approach is not too distant. The data are supportive, and further research is warranted to strengthen the approach.

REFERENCES

1. Hudis C. Trastuzumab – mechanism of action and use in clinical practice. N Engl J Med 2007;357(1): 39–51.
2. Hayes DF, Thor AD, Dressler LG, et al. HER2 and response to paclitaxel in node-positive breast cancer. N Engl J Med 2007;357(15):1496–506.
3. Krause DS, Van Etten RA. Tyrosine kinase as targets for cancer therapy. N Engl J Med 2005;353(2):172–87.
4. Innocenti F, Undevia SD, Lyer L, et al. Genetic variants in the UDP-glucuronosyltransferase 1A1 gene predict the risk of severe neutropenia of irinotecan. J Clin Oncol 2004;22:1382–8.
5. Cote JF, Kirzin S, Kramar A, et al. UGT1A1 polymorphism can predict hematologic toxicity in patients treated with irinotecan. Clin Cancer Res 2007;13: 3269–75.
6. Mallal S, Phillips E, Carosi G, et al. HLA-B*5701 screening for hypersensitivity to abacavir. N Engl J Med 2008;358:568–79.
7. Link E, Parish S, Armitage J, et al. SEARCH Collaborative Group. SLCO1B1 variants and statin-induced myopathy–a genomewide study. N Engl J Med 2008;359(8):789–99.
8. Herman D, Locatelli I, Grabnar I, et al. Influence of CYP2C9 polymorphisms, demographic factors and concomitant drug therapy on warfarin metabolism and maintenance dose. Pharmacogenomics J 2005;5(3):193–202.
9. Schwarz UI, Ritchie MD, Bradford Y, et al. Genetic determinants of response to warfarin during initial anticoagulation. N Engl J Med 2008;358:999–1008.
10. Sotoodehnia N, Siscorick DS, Vatta M, et al. β-2 Adrenergic receptor genetic variants and risk of sudden cardiac death. Circulation 2006;113(15): 1818–20.
11. Rampersaud E, Damcott CM, Fu M, et al. Identification of novel candidate genes for type 2 diabetes from a genome-wide association scan in the Old Order Amish: evidence for replication from diabetes-related quantitative traits and from independent populations. Diabetes 2007;56:3053–62.
12. Saxena R, Voight BF, Lyssenko V, et al. Genome-wide association analysis identifies loci for type 2 diabetes and triglyceride levels. Science 2007;316: 1331–6.
13. Sladek R, Rocheleau G, Rung J, et al. A genome-wide association study identifies novel risk loci for type 2 diabetes. Nature 2007;445:881–5.
14. Wellcome Trust Case Control Consortium. Genome-wide association study of 14,000 cases of seven common diseases and 3,000 shared controls. Nature 2007;447:661–78.
15. Kathiresan S, Manning AK, Demissie S, et al. A genome-wide association study for blood lipid phenotypes in the Framingham Heart Study. BMC Med Genet 2007;8(Suppl 1):S17.
16. Shearman AM, Ordovas JM, Cupples LA, et al. Evidence for a gene influencing the TG/HDL-C ratio on chromosome 7q32,3-qter: a genome-wide scan in the Framingham Study. Hum Mol Genet 2000;9: 1315–20.
17. Peacock JM, Arnett DK, Atwood LD, et al. On behalf of the Investigators of the NHLBI Family Heart Study. Genome scan for quantitative trait loci linked to high-density lipoprotein cholesterol. The NHLBI Family Heart Study. Arterioscler Thromb Vasc Biol 2001; 21:1823–8.

18. O'Donnell CJ, Cupples LA, D'Agostino RB, et al. Genome-wide association study for subclinical atherosclerosis in major arterial territories in the NHLBI's Framingham Heart Study. BMC Med Genet 2007;8(Suppl 1):S4.

19. Samani NJ, Erdmann J, Hall AS, et al. Genomewide association analysis of coronary artery disease. N Engl J Med 2007;357(5):443–53.

20. Lloyd-Jones D, Adams R, Carnethon M, et al. Heart disease and stroke statistics update. Circulation 2009;119:e21–181.

21. Ezekowitz JA, Kaul P, Bakal JA, et al. Declining in-hospital mortality and increasing heart failure incidence in elderly patients with first myocardial infarction. J Am Coll Cardiol 2009;53:13–20.

22. Liggett SB, Mialet-Perez J, Thaneemit-Chen S, et al. A polymorphism within a conserved beta(1)-adrenergic receptor motif alters cardiac function and beta-blocker response in human heart failure. Proc Natl Acad Sci U S A 2006;103:11288–93.

23. de Groote P, Helbecque N, Lamblin N, et al. Association between beta-1 and beta-2 adrenergic receptor gene polymorphisms and the response to beta-blockade in patients with stable congestive heart failure. Pharmacogenet Genomics 2005;15:137–42.

24. Terra SG, Hamilton KK, Pauly DF, et al. Beta1-adrenergic receptor polymorphisms and left ventricular remodeling changes in response to β-blocker therapy. Pharmacogenet Genomics 2005;15:227–34.

25. Rochais F, Vilardaga JP, Nikolaev V, et al. Real-time optical recording of β1-adrenergic receptor activation reveals supersensitivity of the Arg389 variant to carvedilol. J Clin Invest 2007;117(1):229–35.

26. Lindenfeld JL, Plehn JF, Liggett SB, et al. Different patterns of LVEF/remodeling and clinical endpoint effects of bucindolol in beta-1 389 Arg/Gly genotypes. J Card Fail 2008;14(6 Suppl 1):S40.

27. Lindenfeld JL, Liggett SB, Plehn JF, et al. Ischemic cardiomyopathy response to bucindolol may be differentially influenced by beta-1 389 Arg/Gly and alpha-2c genotypes. J Card Fail 2008;14(6 Suppl 1):S77.

28. Mason DA, Moore JD, Green SA, et al. A gain-of-function polymorphism in a G-protein coupling domain of the human beta1-adrenergic receptor. J Biol Chem 1999;274:12670–4.

29. Mialet Perez J, Rathz DA, Petrashevskaya NN, et al. Beta 1-adrenergic receptor polymorphisms confer differential function and predisposition to heart failure. Nat Med 2003;9:1300–5.

30. Sehnert AJ, Daniels SE, Elashoff M, et al. Lack of association between adrenergic receptor genotypes and survival in heart failure patients treated with carvedilol or metoprolol. J Am Coll Cardiol 2008;52:644–51.

31. White H, deBoer RA, Maqbool A, et al. An evaluation of the beta-1 adrenergic receptor Arg389Gly polymorphism in individuals with heart failure: a MERIT-HF sub-study. Eur J Heart Fail 2003;5:463–8.

32. Domanski M, Kraus-Steinrauf H, Massie M, et al. A comparative analysis of the results from 4 trials of beta-blocker therapy for heart failure: BEST, CIBIS-II, MERIT-HF, and COPERNICUS. J Card Fail 2003;9(5):354–63.

33. Walsh R, Farmer R, Kelly M, et al. Human myocardial b1 389 Arg/Arg adrenergic receptors exhibit a propensity for constitutively active, high affinity agonist binding and are selectively inactivated by bucindolol [abstract]. J Card Fail 2008;14(6):S8.

34. Bristow MB, Krause-Steinrauf H, Nuzzo R, et al. Effect of baseline or changes in adrenergic activity on clinical outcomes in the b-blocker evaluation of survival trial. Circulation 2004;110:1437–42.

35. Magnusson Y, Levin M, Eggertsen R, et al. Ser49Gly of β1-adrenergic receptor is associated with effective β-blocker dose in dilated cardiomyopathy. Clin Pharmacol Ther 2005;78:221–31.

36. Forleo C, Sorrentino S, Guida P, et al. β1- and β2-adrenergic receptor polymorphisms affect susceptibility to idiopathic dilated cardiomyopathy. J Cardiovasc Med (Hagerstown) 2007;8(8):589–95.

37. Shin J, Lobmeyer M, Gong Y, et al. Relation of β2-adrenoceptor haplotype to risk of death and heart transplantation in patients with heart failure. Am J Cardiol 2007;99(2):250–5.

38. McNamara DM, Tam SW, Sabolinski ML, et al. Aldosterone synthase promoter polymorphism predicts outcome in African Americans with heart failure. J Am Coll Cardiol 2006;48:1277–82.

39. de Denus S, Zakrzewski-Jakubiak M, Dube MP, et al. Effects of AGTR1 A1166C gene polymorphism in patients with heart failure treated with candesartan. Ann Pharmacother 2008;42:925–32.

40. Kurland L, Melhus H, Karlsson J, et al. Polymorphisms in the angiotensinogen and angiotensin II type 1 receptor gene are related to change in left ventricular mass during antihypertensive treatment: results from the Swedish Irbesartan Left Ventricular Hypertrophy Investigation versus Atenolol (SILVHIA) trial. J Hypertens 2002;20:657–63.

41. Cicoira M, Rossi A, Bonapace S, et al. Effects of ACE gene insertion/deletion polymorphism on response to spironolactone in patients with chronic heart failure. Am J Med 2004;116:657–61.

42. Agerholm-Larsen B, Nordestgaard B, Tybjaerg-Hansen A. ACE gene polymorphism in cardiovascular disease: meta analysis of small and large studies. Arterioscler Thromb Vasc Biol 2000;20:484–92.

43. McNamara DM, Holubkov R, Janosko K, et al. Pharmacogenetic interactions between beta blocker therapy and the angiotensin converting enzyme deletion polymorphism in patients with congestive heart failure. Circulation 2001;103:1644–8.

44. McNamara DM, Holubkov R, Postava L, et al. Pharmacogenetic interactions between ACE inhibitor

therapy and the angiotensin-converting enzyme deletion polymorphism in patients with congestive heart failure. J Am Coll Cardiol 2004;44:2019–26.

45. de Groote P, Helbecque N, Lamblin N. Beta-adrenergic receptor blockade and the angiotensin-converting enzyme deletion polymorphism in patients with chronic heart failure. Eur J Heart Fail 2004;6(1):17–21.

46. Schieffer B. ACE gene polymorphism and coronary artery disease: a question of persuasion or statistical confusion? Arterioscler Thromb Vasc Biol 2000; 20:281.

47. Belardinelli R, Georgiou D, Cianci G, et al. Randomized, controlled trial of long-term moderate exercise training in chronic heart failure: effects on functional capacity, quality of life, and clinical outcome. Circulation 1999;99(9):1173–82.

48. Whellan DJ, O'Connor CM, Lee KL, et al. HF-ACTION Trial Investigators. Heart failure and a controlled trial investigating outcomes of exercise training (HF-ACTION): design and rationale. Am Heart J 2007;153(2):201–11.

49. Eisenach JH, Barnes SA, Pike TL, et al. Arg16/Gly β2-adrenergic receptor polymorphism alters the cardiac output response to isometric exercise. J Appl Physiol 2005;99:1776–81.

50. Trombetta I, Batalha L, Rondon M, et al. Gly16 + Glu27 β2-adrenoceptor polymorphisms cause increased forearm blood flow responses to mental stress and handgrip in humans. J Appl Physiol 2005;98:787–94.

51. McCole S, Shuldiner A, Brown M, et al. β2- and β3-Adrenergic receptor polymorphisms and exercise hemodynamics in postmenopausal women. J Appl Physiol 2004;96:526–30.

52. Wagoner L, Craft L, Singh B, et al. Polymorphisms of the β2-adrenergic receptor determine exercise capacity in patients with heart failure. Circ Res 2000;86:834–40.

53. Kritchevsky S, Nicklas B, Visser M, et al. Angiotensin-converting enzyme insertion/deletion genotype, exercise, and physical decline. JAMA 2005; 294(6):691–8.

54. Abraham M, Olson L, Joyner M, et al. Angiotensin-converting enzyme genotype modulates pulmonary function and exercise capacity in treated patients with congestive stable heart failure. Circulation 2002;106:1794–9.

55. Wieneke H, Naber C, Piaszek L, et al. Better identification of patients who benefit from implantable cardioverter defibrillators by genotyping the G protein β3 subunit (GNB3) C825T polymorphism. Basic Res Cardiol 2006;101(5):447–51.

56. Chemello D, Rohde L, Pimentel M. Role of genetic polymorphisms to predict appropriate therapies in patients with implantable cardioverter defibrillators. J Card Fail 2008;14(6 Suppl 1):S62.

57. Rogers J, Robinson S, Khanna A, et al. Transforming growth factor-β polymorphisms and prediction of clinical outcome with prophylactic defibrillator implantation in chronic heart failure. Circulation 2007;116(Suppl 2):S635.

Reporting of Clinical Trials: Publication, Authorship, and Trial Registration

Raphael E. Bonita, MD, ScM[a],*, Suzanne Adams, RN, MPH[b],
David J. Whellan, MD, MHS[c]

KEYWORDS
- Publication • Authorship • Ghostwriting
- Clinical trial reporting

ASSIGNING AUTHORSHIP: THE PROBLEMS AT HAND

A major criterion for advancement in academic and research careers is the number and quality of publications that one has authored; a researcher's publication record is an important consideration in hiring and promotion decisions. It is also an important factor in securing funding, as the totality of a researcher's publications is seen as a measure of productivity.[1] Assigning manuscript authorship in biomedical literature can be a complex topic and a potentially contentious issue among the parties involved, where decisions may be vulnerable to inappropriate designation that could lead to allegations of misconduct. Prior to some of the controversies discussed in recent peer-reviewed clinical trials literature, relevant areas of concern were described by multidisciplinary researchers in the social sciences, including the following[2]:

1. What specific criteria should be met by an author named on the manuscript byline?
2. What criteria are used to determine the ordering of authors?
3. What other means are available to acknowledge an individual's involvement in the project or contribution to the manuscript?
4. How should honorary authorship, that is, named authors who have not satisfied criteria for authorship, best be managed?
5. How should ghost authorship (active participants in preparation of a manuscript but not listed on the byline) be managed?

Honorary and ghost authorships can be particularly prevalent in the medical literature. A 1998 *JAMA* review found evidence of honorary authorship and ghost authors present in 11% of the medical journals examined.[3] Just 4 years later, a similar study of the *Cochrane Reviews* noted a prevalence of 39% and 9%, respectively.[4]

One criticism of honorary or ghost authorship practices concerns the potential power inequity between senior and junior researchers. Junior researchers may feel obligated or may perceive a benefit from extending honorary authorship to more experienced researchers on a paper to enhance the chances of acceptance into a journal.[5] Senior researchers may view the contributions of the junior researchers as limited to the completion

The authors have nothing to disclose.

[a] Division of Cardiology, Jefferson Medical College, Jefferson Heart Institute, 925 Chestnut Street, Philadelphia, PA 19107, USA
[b] Division of Cardiology, Clinical Outcomes Research and Education, Jefferson Coordinating Center for Clinical Research, Jefferson Medical College, 1015 Chestnut Street, Suite 317, Philadelphia, PA 19107, USA
[c] Division of Cardiology, Department of Medicine, Clinical Outcomes Research and Education, Jefferson Coordinating Center for Clinical Research, Jefferson Medical College, Thomas Jefferson University, 1015 Chestnut Street, Suite 317, Philadelphia, PA 19107, USA
* Corresponding author.
E-mail address: Raphael.Bonita@jefferson.edu

Heart Failure Clin 7 (2011) 561–567
doi:10.1016/j.hfc.2011.06.009

of experiments and data acquisition while not recognizing a valuable contribution of data interpretation.[2] Even when the junior investigator may have met the criteria for authorship and written significant portions of a manuscript, the senior investigator may not acknowledge the contributions and grant an appropriate place in the byline.

It is certainly apparent that concerns regarding honorary and ghost authorship practices in the publication of pharmaceutical and device industry-sponsored studies have increased in the last 10 to 15 years. Previously, the use of journal publications to promote products to the medical community was a fairly common and generally accepted practice, or was unacknowledged or unrecognized by reviewers and readers. However, by the early 2000s specific exposés of various deceptive industry practices designed to enhance marketing and promote sales of certain drugs began to reach professionals and eventually the public at large. The practices included targeted funding for research investigators and strategic educational support, often through unrestricted educational grants. In the case of gabapentin, for example, medical communication companies were paid to develop and publish articles for the peer-reviewed medical literature.[6] Eventually, the practice of industry-generated ghostwriting resulted in an increased number of civil lawsuits (both individual and class action). These trials ultimately provided access to internal industry documents whereby additional evidence of questionable practices could be reviewed and described. A 2008 substantive review of guest authorship and ghostwriting associated with rofecoxib became one of the most widely acknowledged series of financial manipulations between industry and academia.[7] Subsequently, in 2009 the Institute of Medicine recommended that academic medical centers adopt policies to prohibit faculty ghostwriting.[8] However, a 2010 review of 50 United States centers reported that only half had indeed published policies on authorship or ghostwriting.[9]

EXISTING GUIDELINES FOR AUTHORSHIP

Determining who will be listed on the byline as an author can be a complex and contentious issue for the parties involved. In general, authorship should be discussed in the beginnings of any project among the researchers to provide time for negotiation and resolve disputes with any part of the process.[2] Authorship should be reserved for those individuals who contribute significantly to the research project at hand. The determination of what contributions to the manuscript meet the threshold for authorship is not always clear, but one series of potential tasks that may be considered in determining authorship in the allied health professions is included in **Table 1**.[1]

The International Committee of Medical Journal Editors (ICMJE), a working group of general medical journals, developed authorship guidelines to assist prospective authors in the appropriate and ethical assignment of authorship. The ICMJE defines an author as "making a significant contribution to the manuscript" and strongly recommends that the authors be able to identify those responsible for each aspect of the paper. Authorship should thus be based on the following criteria: (1) significant contribution to study or project design and analysis or interpretation of the data; (2) writing and/or revising the manuscript; (3) the authors must finally approve the manuscript at hand. A contributing researcher would have to satisfy all 3 criteria to be considered an author on the accepted version of the paper. The ICMJE would not consider more remote activities such as providing funding support or generalized supervision as sufficient to merit authorship inclusion.

Regarding authorship in a multicenter trial, the investigating group should identify those directly responsible for the preparation and submission of the manuscript, and these individuals should meet the ICMJE criteria for authorship listed above. On a manuscript submission from an investigator group, the corresponding author should indicate the preferred citation, and identify the individual authors and the group name. All members of the group should satisfy the criteria for authorship. Individuals who not meet any of the criteria for authorship should be listed as contributors in the acknowledgment section of the paper. For instance, a participant whose only task was to collect data or to assist in the writing of the manuscript, or who was involved in a particular technical aspect of the project should generally not be listed as an author but should be acknowledged as a contributor.[10] To expand on full disclosure of authorship criteria, some propose that in addition to a substantial intellectual investment, named authors be required to list their particular contributions to the project. The researchers would select from a predefined list of tasks that best reflected their involvement, or could describe in their own words how they contributed to the manuscript. This process has been adopted by some but not all biomedical journals. Concerns over the reliability and validity of the contributor lists, and that the lists themselves can be viewed as somewhat "wasted" space at the end of the article, have been cited as some of the perceived drawbacks to this practice.[11,12]

Table 1
Actions and intellectual tasks considered for authorship among various groups

Bourbonniere et al[1]	CanChild Guidelines	National Psychosis Research Framework	ICMJE
Origination of study idea	Substantial intellectual contribution to the project involving study design	Principal investigators from each site must provide a written agreement on the data and authorship assignment policy early on in the process to avoid potential conflicts	Significant contribution to study or project design
Developed the study design			Significant contribution to study or project analysis plan
Wrote the grant	Substantial intellectual contribution to the project involving data interpretation		Significant contribution to study or project data interpretation
Interviewed study subjects			Writing the manuscript
Managed project data			Editing the manuscript
Interpreted results	Significant contribution to the writing of the manuscript	Authorship should reflect significant contributions to the study	Author approval of the manuscript
Wrote the manuscript			
Revised/edited the manuscript	Official approval of the final version of the paper	Development of manuscripts including study design, data interpretation, writing, and revisions	
Supervised data analyses	Full responsibility for the finished manuscript	Investigators that do not meet criteria for authorship of the study can be named in the acknowledgment section of the paper	
Provided technical support		Prior to publication, authors should offer written approval of the contents and final version of the manuscript	
Approved the final draft before submission		Papers using data from other sites should acknowledge the entire research group	

There are alternatives to the ICMJE models to guide the assignment of authorship for publication. The CanChild Center for Childhood Disability Research methods (a modification of the ICMJE criteria) also have broad applicability for biomedical research publication. The CanChild guidelines require that the following criteria be satisfied: (1) substantial intellectual contribution to the project involving study design or data interpretation; (2) significant contribution to the actual writing or revision of the manuscript; (3) official approval of the final version of the paper; and (4) full responsibility for the finished manuscript. While these provide a more detailed description of the contributions necessary for authorship, they are somewhat limited in scope and applicability in more complex scenarios such as determining authorship in multi-center clinical trials.

The National Psychosis Research Framework also established guidelines for defining authorship involving multicentered research trials.[13] A summary of the salient points from these guidelines states:

1. Principal investigators from each site must provide a written agreement on the data and authorship assignment policy early on in the process to avoid potential conflicts
2. Authorship should reflect significant contributions to the study and development of manuscripts including study design, data interpretation, writing, and revisions

3. Investigators that do not meet criteria for authorship of the study can be named in the acknowledgment section of the paper
4. Prior to publication, authors should offer written approval of the contents and final version of the manuscript at hand
5. Papers using data from other sites should acknowledge the entire research group.

The National Psychosis Research Framework provides direction in terms of handling authorship assignment issues and stresses when research is multicentered, but this is limited in scope in providing specific details on how to assign authorship when multiple secondary manuscripts develop from the original project idea.

In addition to criteria for determining authorship, ordering in the author block of the manuscript can also be a complex and debatable issue for the parties involved; none of the aforementioned guidelines address the issue of ordering. Traditional practices designate the lead author (the first listed) as the individual making the greatest contribution to the project. The last author position has traditionally been reserved for the most senior researcher of the project.[14]

AUTHORSHIP ASSIGNMENT IN MULTICENTER CLINICAL TRIALS

When authors from several centers participate in manuscript preparation, listing the authors in a manner that is consistent with their respective contribution to the research project becomes a more complicated issue. Several groups have developed various weighting systems based on the assignment of points for contributing to various aspects of the research project and manuscript production. The authors can be ranked according to the number of points each has accumulated, and the author order is then based on this point system.[5,15,16]

PROPOSED MODELS

A more involved algorithm for authorship assignment regarding the process of assigning authorship in HF-ACTION was recently published by Whellan and colleagues.[17] The HF-ACTION (Heart Failure: A Controlled Trial Investigating Outcomes of Exercise Training) trial (clinicaltrials.gov registration number: NCT00047437) was a multicentered trial that randomized symptomatic heart failure patients with left ventricular systolic dysfunction to either formal exercise training or standard care.[18] The study involved 98 investigators from 82 regional centers (from the United States, Canada, and France). Within HF-ACTION, the process of determining authorship involved two steps: (1) collecting

personnel interests regarding potential future manuscripts and (2) ranking site personnel to assign authors. A list of manuscript topics proposed by the HF-ACTION executive committee was circulated to principal investigators, who were then asked to rank their top 5 topics where a score of 1 represented their highest interest (**Fig. 1**). In addition, the principal investigator could select other personnel, coinvestigators, and study coordinators, to rank 5 manuscript topics they might be interested in. The publication committee was then responsible for assigning authorship and authorship position based on the investigator site's score. The site score was based on site-specific metrics that were converted into a score. Site-specific metrics included (1) enrollment, (2) adherence to the exercise regimen, (3) data completion and submission, and (4) general trial operations. The scores for the specific metrics were weighted and summed for a final score (**Fig. 2**). Each clinical trial site was then ranked according to the total number of points. The authors were then determined and the order of authorship established by using the choice of manuscript given by the site's principal investigator. Points were "spent" from each site according to authorship position: 150 points for lead author, 100 points for senior author, and 50 points for co-author. Sites were reranked after each author assignment, and this process continued until all manuscript topics were assigned. Investigators interested in pursuing topics not included in the proposed topic list could submit their own topics. Thus, the HF-ACTION method for identifying authors not only established whether an investigator could be an author but also guided the authorship position based on trial participation.

CLINICAL TRIALS REPORTING: THE IMPORTANCE OF REGISTRATION

Before 2005, registration of clinical trials was not required or commonplace. In an effort to promote transparency and honesty among the research community and with the public regarding appropriate research conduct, the World Health Organization (WHO) set forth an initiative recommending clinical trial registration.[19] In 2005 the ICMJE required clinical trial investigators to enroll in an accepted trial registry (Clinical trials registration: a statement from the ICMJE, available at www.icmje.org). The ICMJE requires that studies meeting the definition of a clinical trial, that is, "any research study that prospectively assigns human participants or groups of humans to one or more health-related interventions to evaluate the effects on health outcomes," be registered in 1 of the 5 existing ICMJE-approved registries or

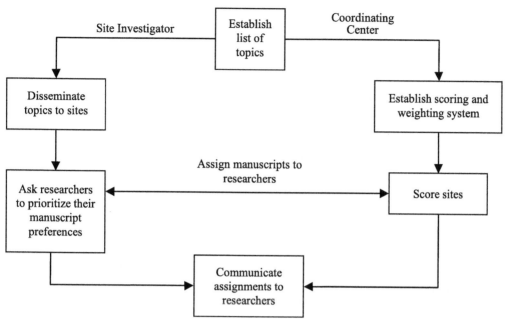

Fig. 1. Flow chart outlining process and tasks developed by the Executive and Publications Committee for establishing authorship in the HF-ACTION study. (*From* Whellan DJ, Ellis SJ, Kraus WE, et al. Method for establishing authorship in a multicenter clinical trial. Ann Intern Med 2009;151:414–20; with permission.)

any registry that participates in the WHO International Clinical Trial Registry Platform.[20] Any clinical trial supported by National Institutes of Health (NIH) funds must be registered no later than 21 days after the enrollment of the first subject.

Further, it is mandated that datasets generated during the duration of the study be made public in the form of summary results via an online database widely accessible to the public. The data are required to be presented to the public in an

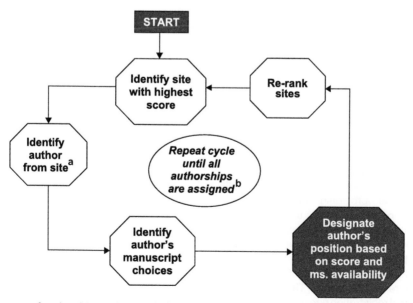

Fig. 2. Assignment of authorship method developed for the HF-ACTION study. [a]Authors include principal investigator, co–principal investigator, and other study personnel. [b]Assign available positions: lead author (first author), senior author (second, third, or last), and co-author (all other positions). Points for assignment are as follows: lead = 150 points, senior = 100 points, and co-author = 50 points. (*From* Whellan DJ, Ellis SJ, Kraus WE, et al. Method for establishing authorship in a multicenter clinical trial. Ann Intern Med 2009;151:416; with permission.)

informative, standardized format. The information that needs to be reported includes, but is not limited to, demographic and baseline data, primary and secondary outcomes, number of patients that dropped out or were excluded from the study, statistical analyses, and contact information for the research group. As of September 2009, researchers responsible for conducting clinical trials are also mandated to report the number and frequency of adverse events that may have occurred in the course of the study. The timeline for reporting the results of a completed study is 12 months after the estimated or actual completion of data collection, whichever comes first. Noncompliance could result in NIH funding being withheld or rescinded, sanctions imposed by the US Food and Drug Administration (FDA), monetary penalties (up to $10,000), and public notices of noncompliance. Similar penalties can be imposed for failure to register.[21]

International guidelines exist, such as the Declaration of Helsinki and CONSORT regarding the ethical requirements for authors and researchers. The Declaration of Helsinki, developed in 1964 and subsequently revised by the World Medical Association, states that researchers are obligated to make available the results of all research studies, whether the study result is negative or positive, again attempting to address the issue of publication bias (www.wma.net). The Consolidated Standards of Reporting Trials Statement (CONSORT), another set of principles for researchers to follow, is intended to improve the reporting of actual trial results. This guideline is composed of a checklist of items that should be used when reporting the trial's design, methods, and outcomes.[22]

This issue is an important one, because those studies that are showing a significant positive result will play a major role in the intervention becoming an accepted therapy. By maintaining a record of all studies prior to results being known, the public and health care community has the opportunity to evaluate new therapies or interventions with greater transparency.

Other important reasons to have clinical trials registered include providing the public/other researchers the opportunity to further analyze the reasons why the respective trial was negative or null, namely poor study design.[23] Further study of these "failed" trials may allow the research community to avoid the situation repeating itself by improving future trial design. The WHO also suggests that trial registration can prevent unnecessary research duplication, improve patient recruitment, enhance collaboration between research groups by making results more accessible, and potentially improve trial design.

Public registries are intended to minimize the impact of publication bias. The ability to evaluate and compare positive trial results (which are more likely to be accepted for publication) with negative or neutral study results of the same therapy allows for a more balanced interpretation of a treatment's efficacy. Clinical trials with favorable results from the FDA were 5 times more likely to be published than negative ones.[24] A recent review of the acceptance rates showed that only 5.3% of all negative studies were accepted for publication.[25]

SUMMARY

Over the past 10 years, repeated exposures of questionable industry practices in manipulating clinical trials data in biomedical publications has weakened the credibility of academic authorship and undercut public confidence in clinical research outcomes to some degree. The requirements for registration and public reporting of research methods and results in the ClinicalTrials.gov registry database provide the most significant transparency practices to date. Practices associated with ghostwriting disclosure have not yet been addressed in such a widespread manner. Guidelines such as those created by ICMJE offer directions for management of authorship; however, additional and more sophisticated strategies will be needed to ensure trust.

REFERENCES

1. Bourbonniere MC, Russell DJ, Goldsmith CH. Authorship issues: one research center's experience with developing author guidelines. Am J Occup Ther 2006;60:111–7.

2. British Sociological Association (1996) BSA guidelines for postgraduate research in sociology, Available at: http://www.britsoc.org.uk/about/postgradres.htm. Accessed August 1, 2010.

3. Flanagin A, Carey LA, Fontanarosa PB, et al. Prevalence of articles with honorary authors and ghost authors in peer-reviewed medical journals. JAMA 1998;280:222–4.

4. Mowatt G, Shirran L, Grimshaw JM, et al. Prevalence of honorary and ghost authorship in Cochrane reviews. JAMA 2002;287:2769–71.

5. Bhopal R, Rankin J, McColl E, et al. The vexed question of authorship: views of researchers in a British medical faculty. BMJ 1997;314:1009–12.

6. Steinman MA, Bero LA, Chren MM, et al. Narrative review: the promotion of gabapentin: an analysis of internal industry documents. Ann Intern Med 2006; 145:284–93.

7. Ross JS, Hill KP, Egilman DS, et al. Guest authorship and ghostwriting in publications related to rofecoxib. JAMA 2008;299:1800–12.

8. Institute of Medicine. Conflict of interest in medical research, education, and practice. (2009). Available at: http://books.nap.edu/openbook.php?record_id=12598. Accessed August 1, 2010.

9. Lacass JR, Leo J. Ghostwriting at elite academic medical centers in the United States. PLoS Med 2010; 7:e1000230. DOI:10.1371/journal.pmed.1000230.

10. International Committee of Medical Journal Editors. Uniform requirements for manuscripts submitted to biomedical journals: writing and editing for biomedical publication (October 2007). Available at: http://www.icmje.org/. Accessed August 26, 2010.

11. Yank V, Rennie D. Disclosure of researcher contributions: a study of original research articles in The Lancet. Ann Intern Med 1999;130:661–70.

12. Savitz DA. What can we infer from author order in epidemiology? Am J Epidemiol 1999;149:401–3.

13. Barker A, Powell RA. Authorship. Guidelines exist on ownership of data and authorship in multicentre collaborations. BMJ 1997;314:1046.

14. Higham NJ. Handbook of writing for the mathematical sciences. Philadelphia: Society for Industrial and Applied Mathematics; 1993.

15. Digiusto E. Equity in authorship: a strategy for assigning credit when publishing. Soc Sci Med 1994; 38:55–8.

16. Ahmed SM, Maurana CA, Engle JA, et al. A method for assigning authorship in multiauthored publications. Fam Med 1997;29:42–4.

17. Whellan DJ, Ellis SJ, Kraus WE, et al. Method for establishing authorship in a multicenter clinical trial. Ann Intern Med 2009;151:414–20.

18. O'Connor CM, Whellan DJ, Lee KL, et al. Efficacy and safety of exercise training in patients with chronic heart failure: HF-ACTION randomized controlled trial. JAMA 2009;301:1439–50.

19. Mandelbaum-Schmid J. The World Health Organization announces new standards for registration of all human medical research, May 19, 2006. Available at: http://www.who.int/mediacentre/news/releases/2006. Accessed June 13, 2011.

20. Laine C, De Angelis C, Delamothe T, et al. Clinical trial registration: looking back and moving ahead. Ann Intern Med 2007;147:275–7.

21. NIH Fact Sheet (10/27/09) on registration at ClinicalTrials.gov under FDAAA 801. Available at: www.prsinfo.clinicaltrials.gov/s801-fact-sheet.pdf. Accessed August 20, 2010.

22. Moher D, Schulz KF, Altman DG. The CONSORT statement: revised recommendations for improving the quality of reports of parallel-group randomised trials. Lancet 2001;357:1191–4.

23. Foote M. Review of current authorship guidelines and the controversy regarding publication of clinical trial data. Biotechnol Annu Rev 2003;9:303–13.

24. Olson CM, Rennie D, Cook D, et al. Publication bias in editorial decision making. JAMA 2002;287:2825–8.

25. Sridharan L, Greenland P. Editorial policies and publication bias: the importance of negative studies. Arch Intern Med 2009;169:1022–3.

Index

Note: Page numbers of article titles are in **boldface** type.

doi:10.1016/S1551-7136(11)00077-8
1551-7136/11/$ – see front matter © 2011 Elsevier Inc. All rights reserved.

heartfailure.theclinics.com

United States Postal Service

Statement of Ownership, Management, and Circulation
(All Periodicals Publications Except Requestor Publications)

1. Publication Title	2. Publication Number	3. Filing Date
Heart Failure Clinics	0 2 5 - 0 5 5	9/16/11

4. Issue Frequency	5. Number of Issues Published Annually	6. Annual Subscription Price
Jan, Apr, July, Oct	4	$207.00

7. Complete Mailing Address of Known Office of Publication (Not printer) (Street, city, county, state, and ZIP+4®)

Elsevier Inc.
360 Park Avenue South
New York, NY 10010-1710

Contact Person
Stephen Bushing

Telephone (Include area code)
215-239-3688

8. Complete Mailing Address of Headquarters or General Business Office of Publisher (Not printer)

Elsevier Inc., 360 Park Avenue South, New York, NY 10010-1710

9. Full Names and Complete Mailing Addresses of Publisher, Editor, and Managing Editor (Do not leave blank)

Publisher (Name and complete mailing address)

Kim Murphy, Elsevier, Inc., 1600 John F. Kennedy Blvd. Suite 1800, Philadelphia, PA 19103-2899

Editor (Name and complete mailing address)

Barbara Cohen-Kligerman, Elsevier, Inc., 1600 John F. Kennedy Blvd. Suite 1800, Philadelphia, PA 19103-2899

Managing Editor (Name and complete mailing address)

Barbara Cohen-Kligerman, Elsevier, Inc., 1600 John F. Kennedy Blvd. Suite 1800, Philadelphia, PA 19103-2899

10. Owner (Do not leave blank. If the publication is owned by a corporation, give the name and address of the corporation immediately followed by the names and addresses of all stockholders owning or holding 1 percent or more of the total amount of stock. If not owned by a corporation, give the names and addresses of the individual owners. If owned by a partnership or other unincorporated firm, give its name and address as well as those of each individual owner. If the publication is published by a nonprofit organization, give its name and address.)

Full Name	Complete Mailing Address
Wholly owned subsidiary of	4520 East-West Highway
Reed/Elsevier, US holdings	Bethesda, MD 20814

11. Known Bondholders, Mortgagees, and Other Security Holders Owning or Holding 1 Percent or More of Total Amount of Bonds, Mortgages, or Other Securities. If none, check box ▶ ☐ None

Full Name	Complete Mailing Address
N/A	

12. Tax Status (For completion by nonprofit organizations authorized to mail at nonprofit rates) (Check one)
The purpose, function, and nonprofit status of this organization and the exempt status for federal income tax purposes:
☐ Has Not Changed During Preceding 12 Months
☐ Has Changed During Preceding 12 Months (Publisher must submit explanation of change with this statement)

PS Form 3526, September 2007 (Page 1 of 3 (Instructions Page 3)) PSN 7530-01-000-9931 PRIVACY NOTICE: See our Privacy policy in www.usps.com

---

13. Publication Title	14. Issue Date for Circulation Data Below
Heart Failure Clinics	July 2011

15. Extent and Nature of Circulation		Average No. Copies Each Issue During Preceding 12 Months	No. Copies of Single Issue Published Nearest to Filing Date
a. Total Number of Copies (Net press run)		536	653
b. Paid Circulation (By Mail and Outside the Mail)	(1) Mailed Outside-County Paid Subscriptions Stated on PS Form 3541. (Include paid distribution above nominal rate, advertiser's proof copies, and exchange copies)	77	74
	(2) Mailed In-County Paid Subscriptions Stated on PS Form 3541 (Include paid distribution above nominal rate, advertiser's proof copies, and exchange copies)		
	(3) Paid Distribution Outside the Mails Including Sales Through Dealers and Carriers, Street Vendors, Counter Sales, and Other Paid Distribution Outside USPS®	21	21
	(4) Paid Distribution by Other Classes Mailed Through the USPS (e.g. First-Class Mail®)		
c. Total Paid Distribution (Sum of 15b (1), (2), (3), and (4))	▶	98	95
d. Free or Nominal Rate Distribution (By Mail and Outside the Mail)	(1) Free or Nominal Rate Outside-County Copies Included on PS Form 3541	61	66
	(2) Free or Nominal Rate In-County Copies Included on PS Form 3541		
	(3) Free or Nominal Rate Copies Mailed at Other Classes Through the USPS (e.g. First-Class Mail)		
	(4) Free or Nominal Rate Distribution Outside the Mail (Carriers or other means)		
e. Total Free or Nominal Rate Distribution (Sum of 15d (1), (2), (3) and (4))	▶	61	66
f. Total Distribution (Sum of 15c and 15e)	▶	159	161
g. Copies not Distributed (See instructions to publishers #4 (page #3))	▶	377	492
h. Total (Sum of 15f and g)	▶	536	653
i. Percent Paid (15c divided by 15f times 100)		61.64%	59.01%

16. Publication of Statement of Ownership
☐ If the publication is a general publication, publication of this statement is required. Will be printed in the October 2011 issue of this publication. ☐ Publication not required

17. Signature and Title of Editor, Publisher, Business Manager, or Owner	Date
Stephen R. Bushing — Inventory/Distribution Coordinator	September 16, 2011

Stephen R. Bushing – Inventory Distribution Coordinator

I certify that all information furnished on this form is true and complete. I understand that anyone who furnishes false or misleading information on this form or who omits material or information requested on the form may be subject to criminal sanctions (including fines and imprisonment) and/or civil sanctions (including civil penalties).

PS Form 3526, September 2007 (Page 2 of 3)

Moving?

Make sure your subscription moves with you!

To notify us of your new address, find your **Clinics Account Number** (located on your mailing label above your name), and contact customer service at:

Email: journalscustomerservice-usa@elsevier.com

800-654-2452 (subscribers in the U.S. & Canada)
314-447-8871 (subscribers outside of the U.S. & Canada)

Fax number: 314-447-8029

Elsevier Health Sciences Division
Subscription Customer Service
3251 Riverport Lane
Maryland Heights, MO 63043

*To ensure uninterrupted delivery of your subscription, please notify us at least 4 weeks in advance of move.

Printed and bound by CPI Group (UK) Ltd, Croydon, CR0 4YY

03/10/2024

01040360-0003